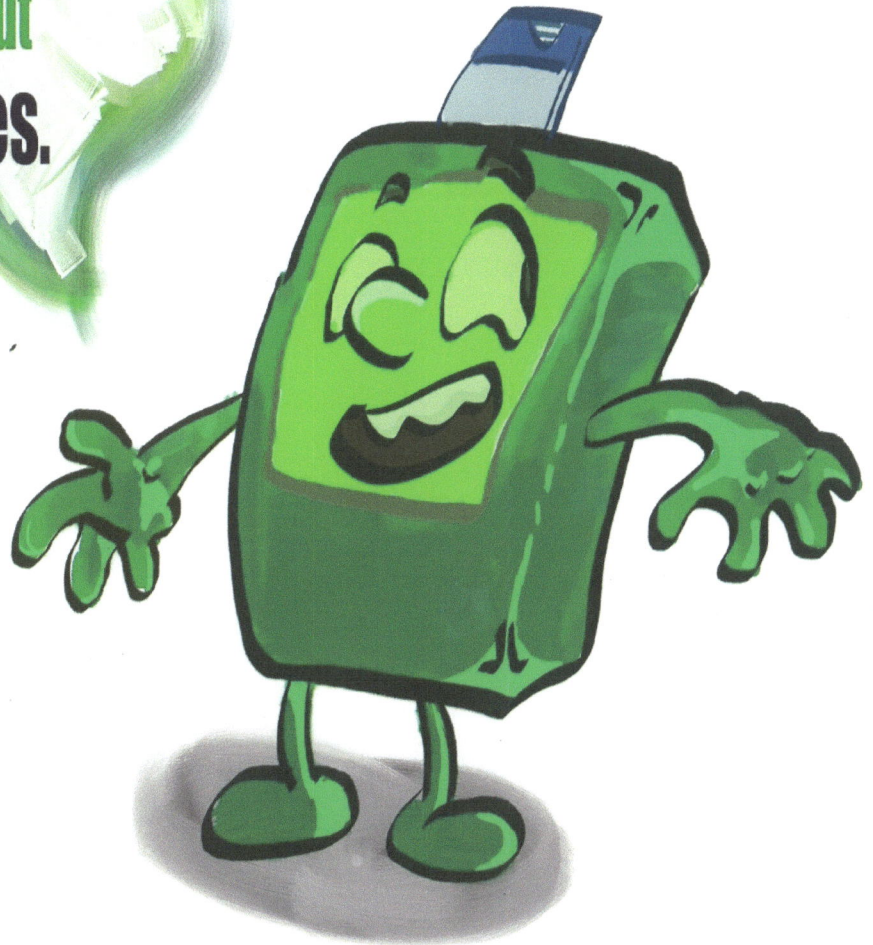

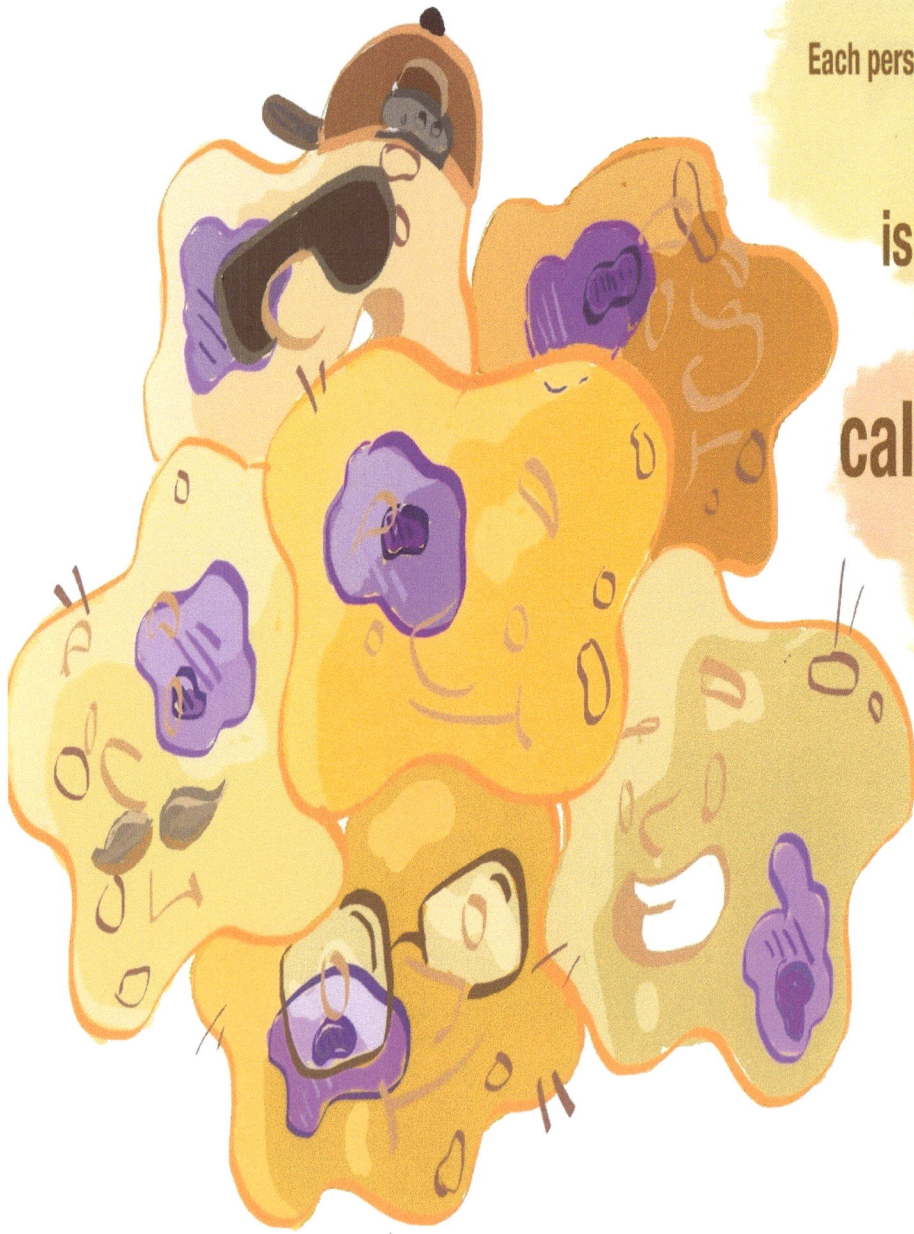

Each person's **body** is made up of **tiny units** called **cells.**

There are many **unique** types of **cells!** Each type has its own **special job.**

Phagocytes swallow harmful germs to keep you healthy.

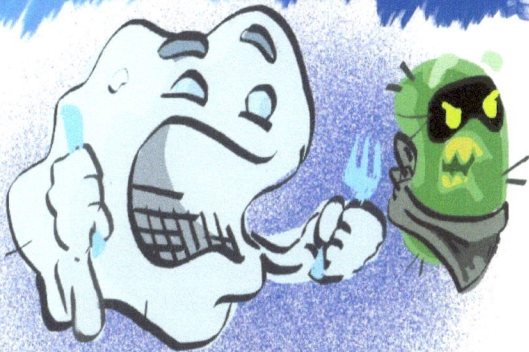

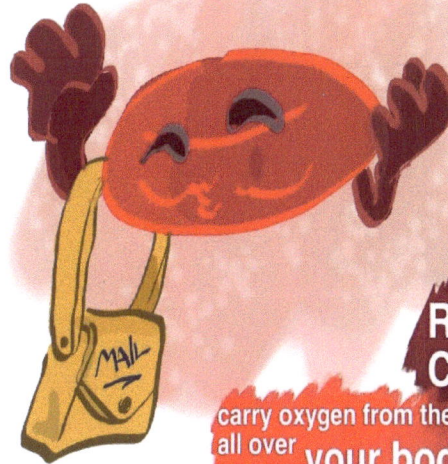

Red Blood Cells carry oxygen from the air you breathe all over **your body.**

Neurons help you **move and feel.**

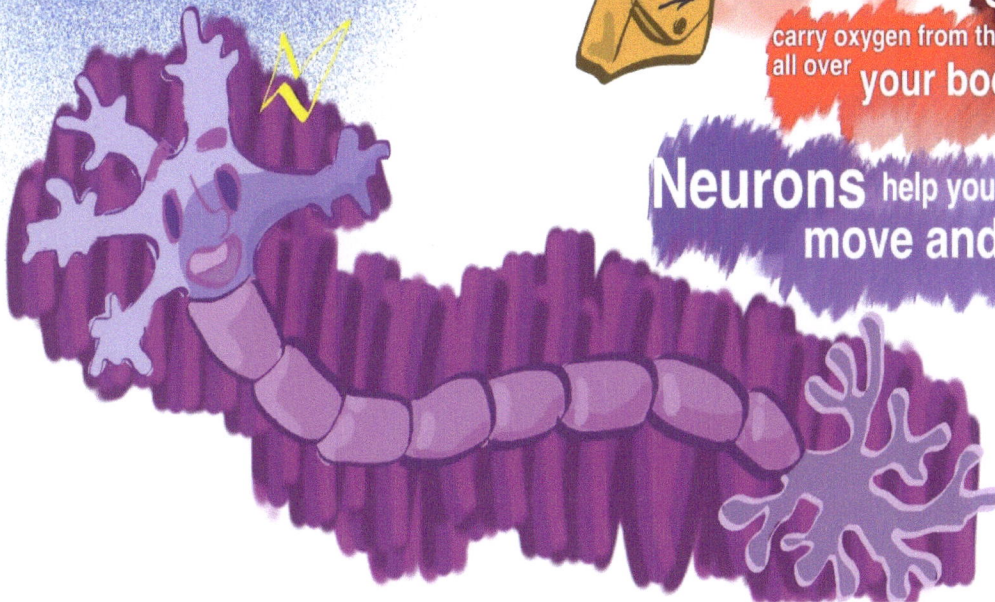

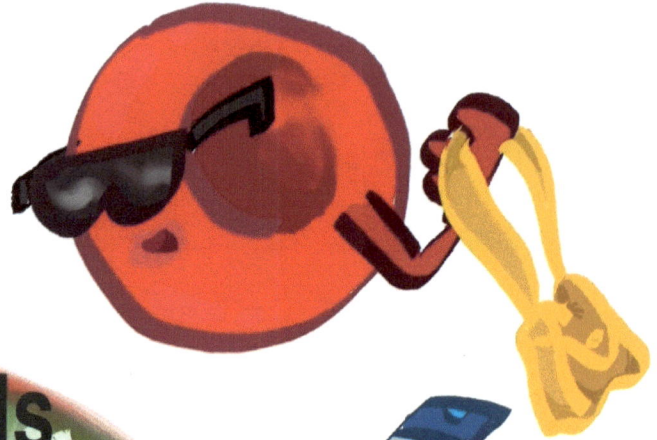

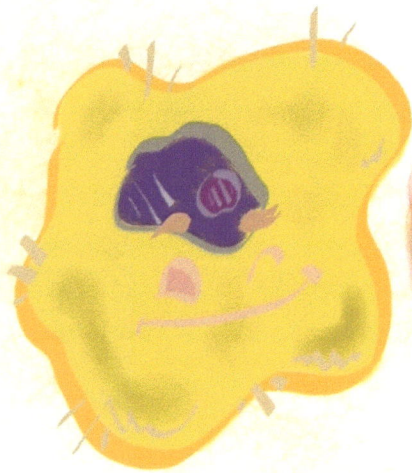

The **cells** in your body all **work very hard** to do their jobs and keep you **healthy!**

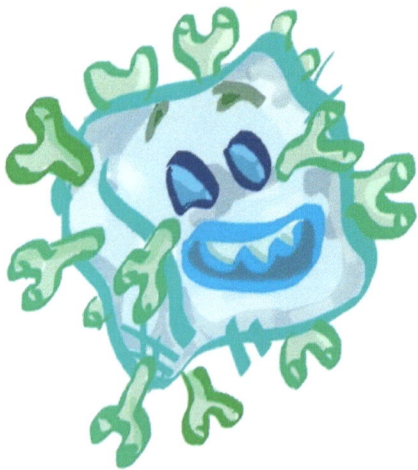

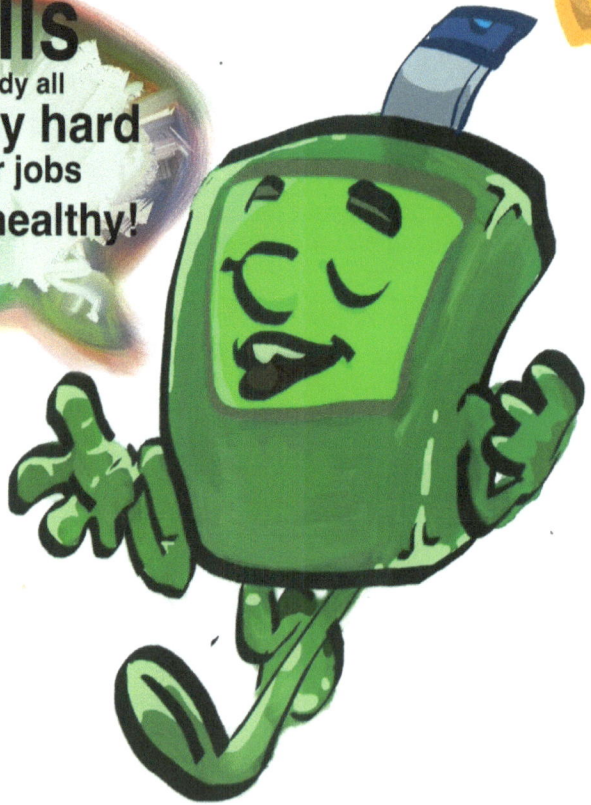

In order to do that, your cells need **fuel** to give them the energy they need to keep running!

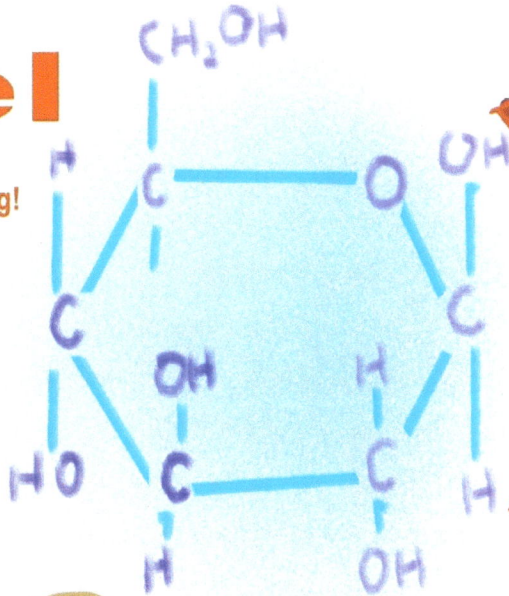

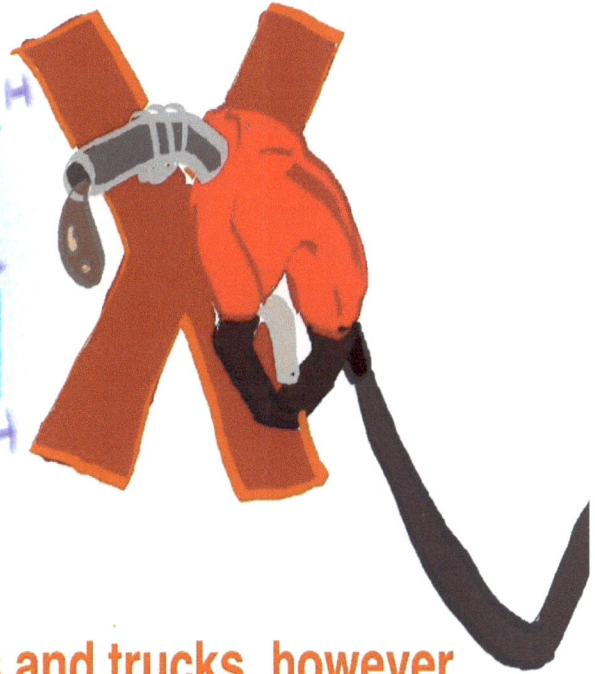

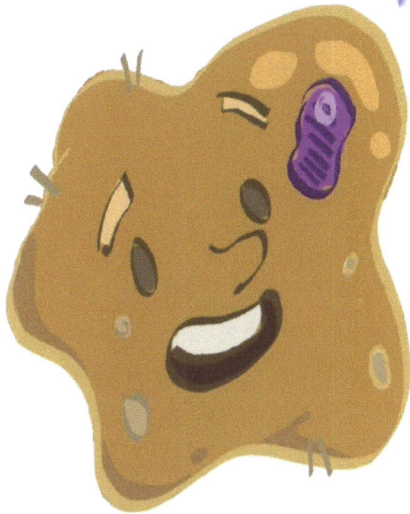

Unlike cars and trucks, however, which use fuels such as gasoline, cells rely on **glucose,** a molecule found in many foods.

Despite how important it is to them, cells can't actually tell when they should take in glucose. In order to get the fuel they need, cells need to be told when it's time to take in glucose.

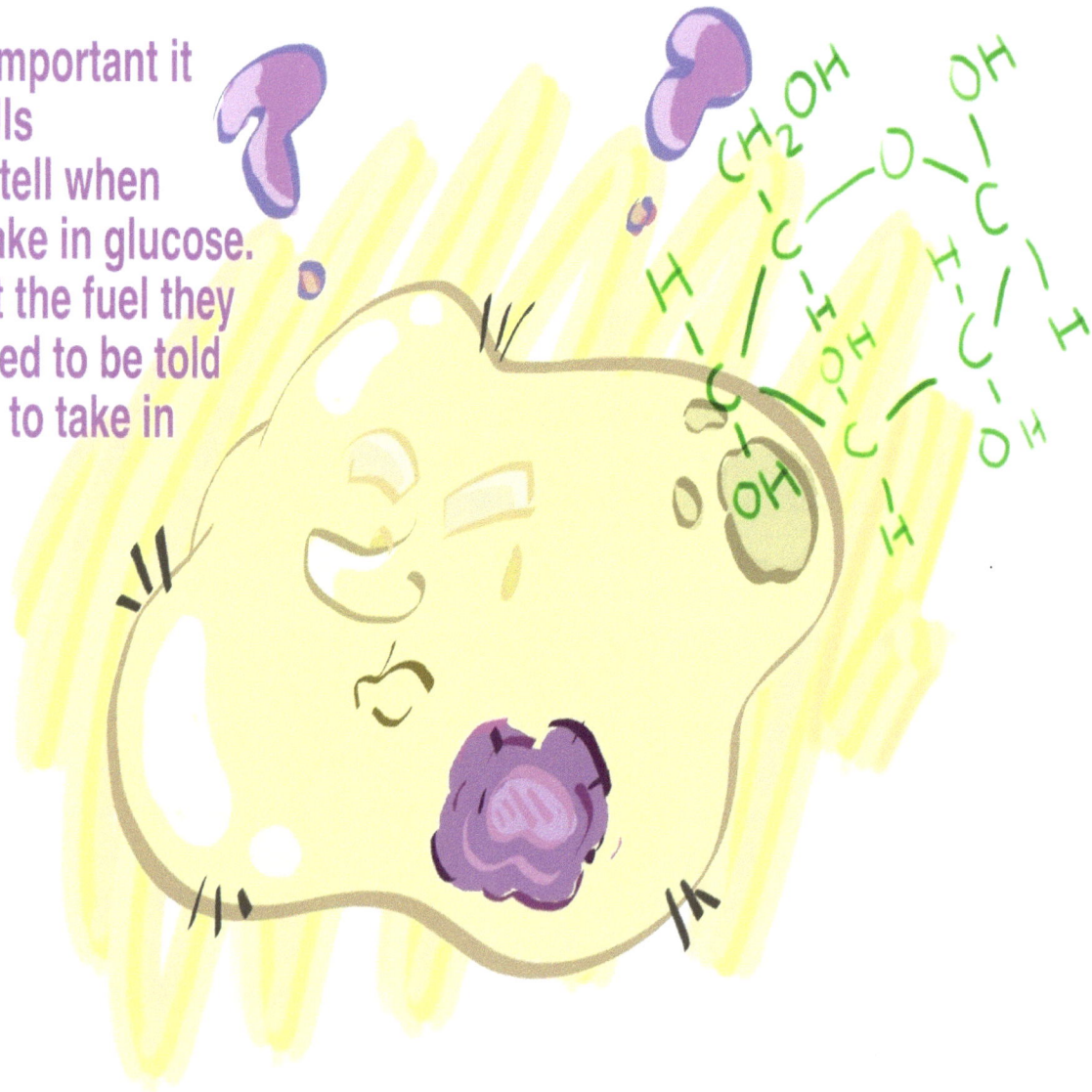

Luckily, the body has an organ whose job is to do just that!

The **pancreas** is a member of the **endocrine** system.

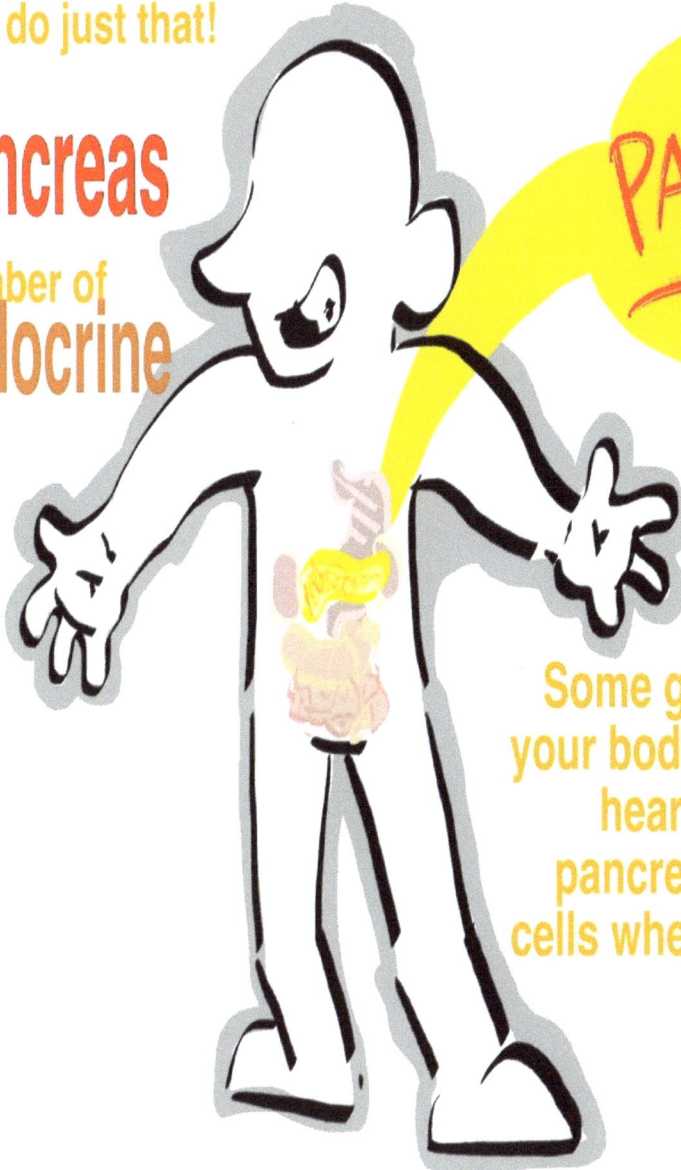

PANCREAS

The endocrine system is a group of glands and organs that send important instructions to cells in the human body!

Some glands and organs help tell your body to grow, or make your heart beat faster, but your pancreas's job is to tell your cells when to take in glucose.

Unlike people, cells can't call, text, or email each other to communicate.

Instead, all endocrine system cells make tiny messengers called hormones to deliver instructions to cells.

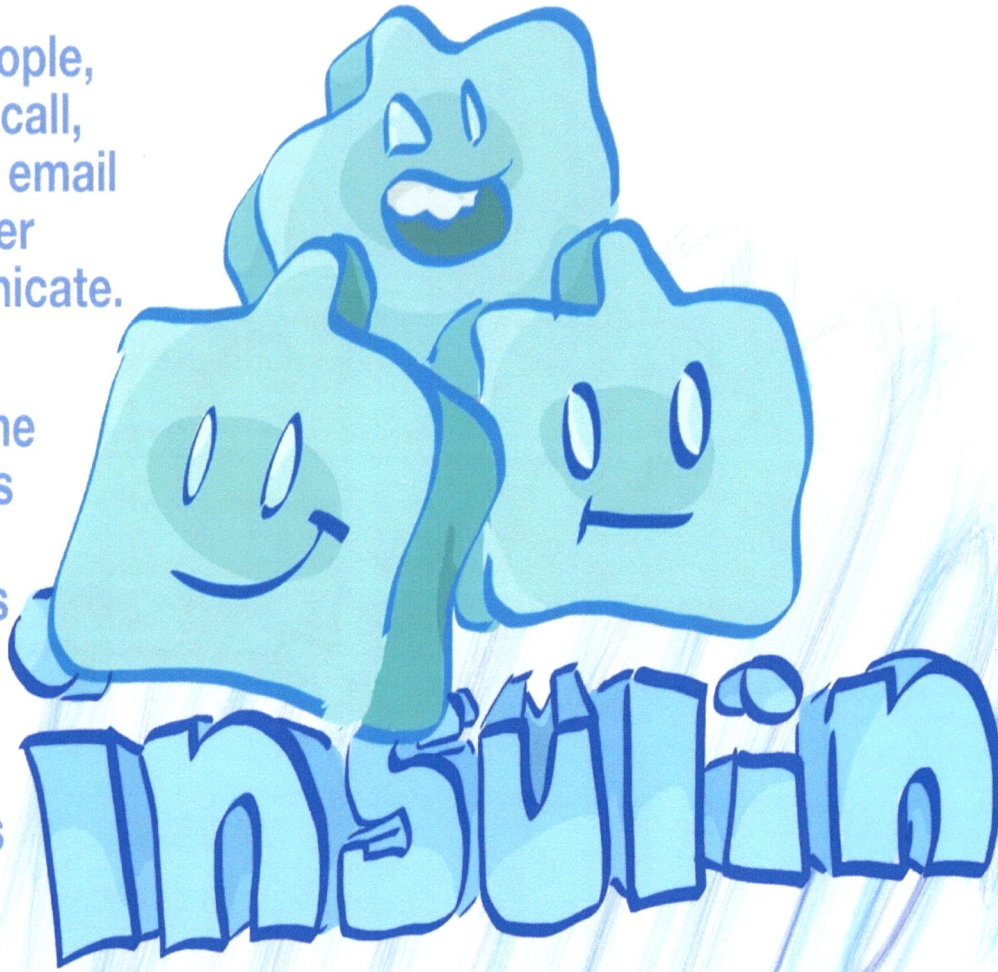

insulin

The pancreas makes the hormone **insulin,** which travels around the body and tells cells to take in glucose.

Insulin connects
to special appendages
on a cell's surface
specially made to fit
insulin called
insulin receptors.
**When insulin
attaches to
insulin
receptors,
it lets cells
know it's time
for them to
take in glucose!**

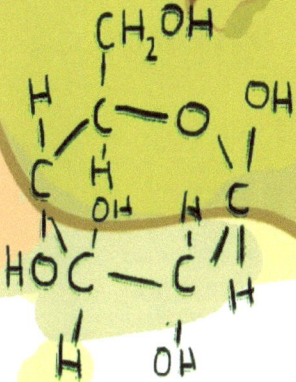

CH_2OH

H C O OH

C H

H OH

HOC C H

H OH

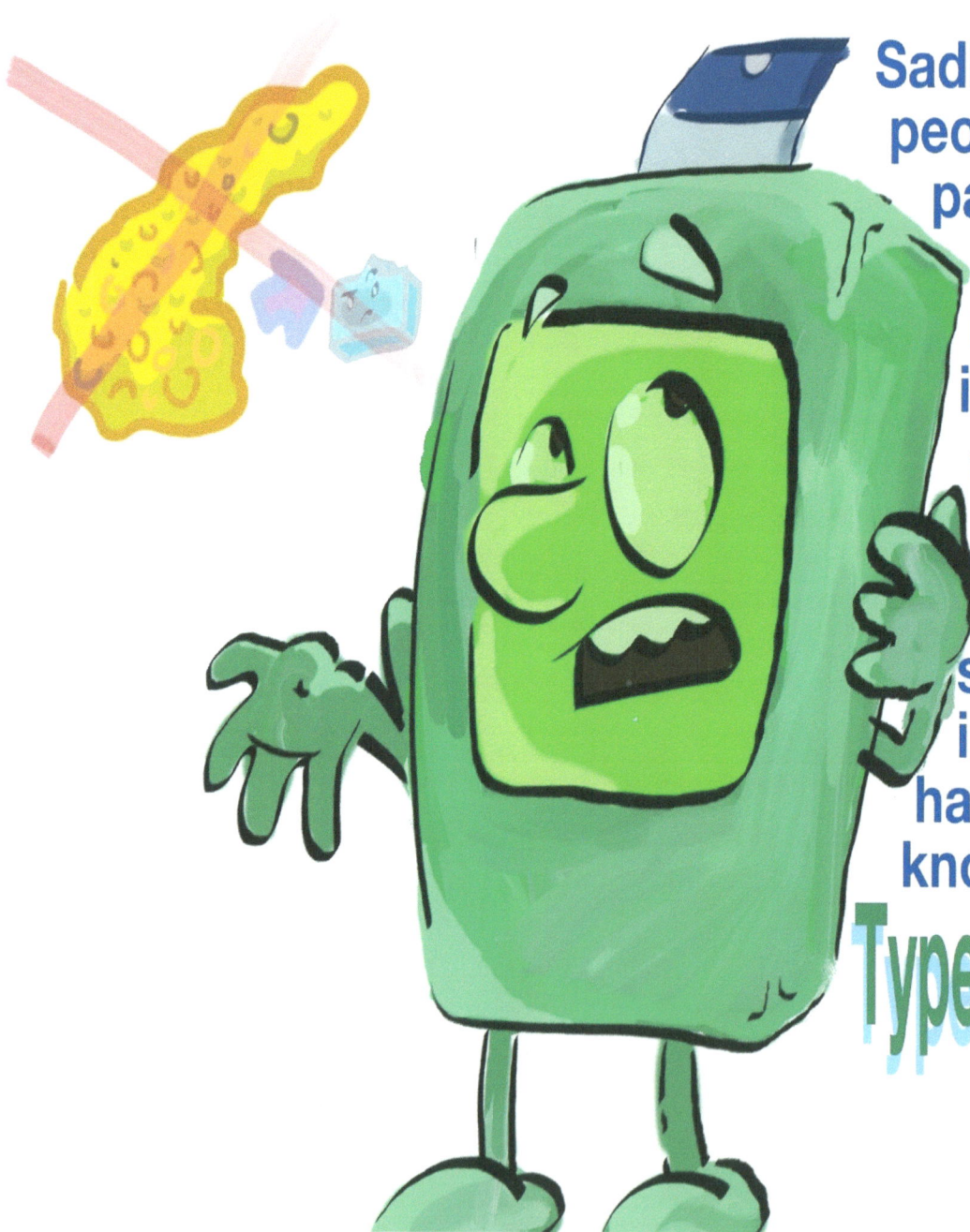

Sadly, some people's pancreases stop making insulin.

When someone's pancreas stops making insulin, they have a condition known as

Type 1 Diabetes

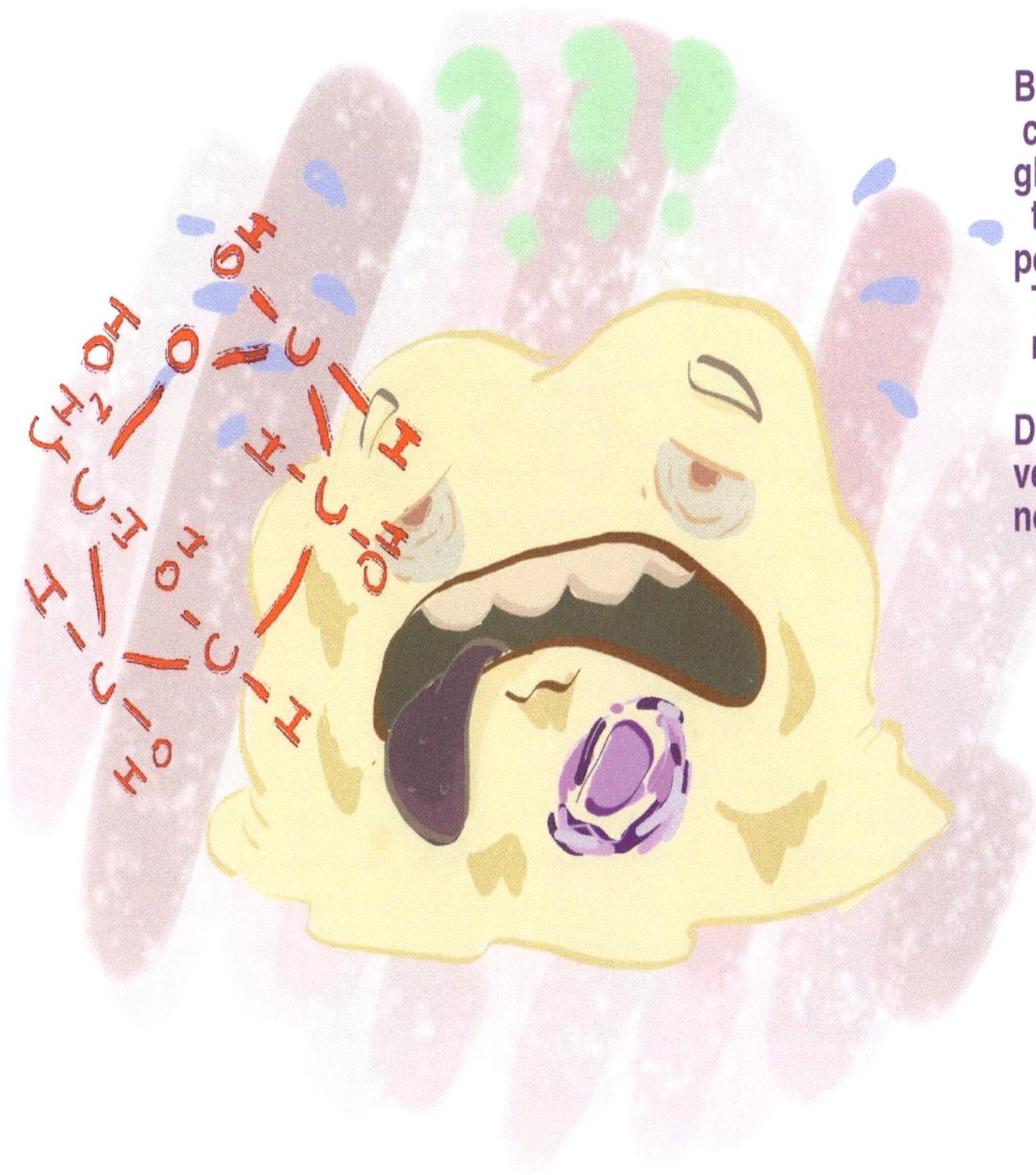

Because their cells can't get the glucose they need to do their jobs, people with Type 1 Diabetes may feel very sick.

Diabetes can be very dangerous if not treated.

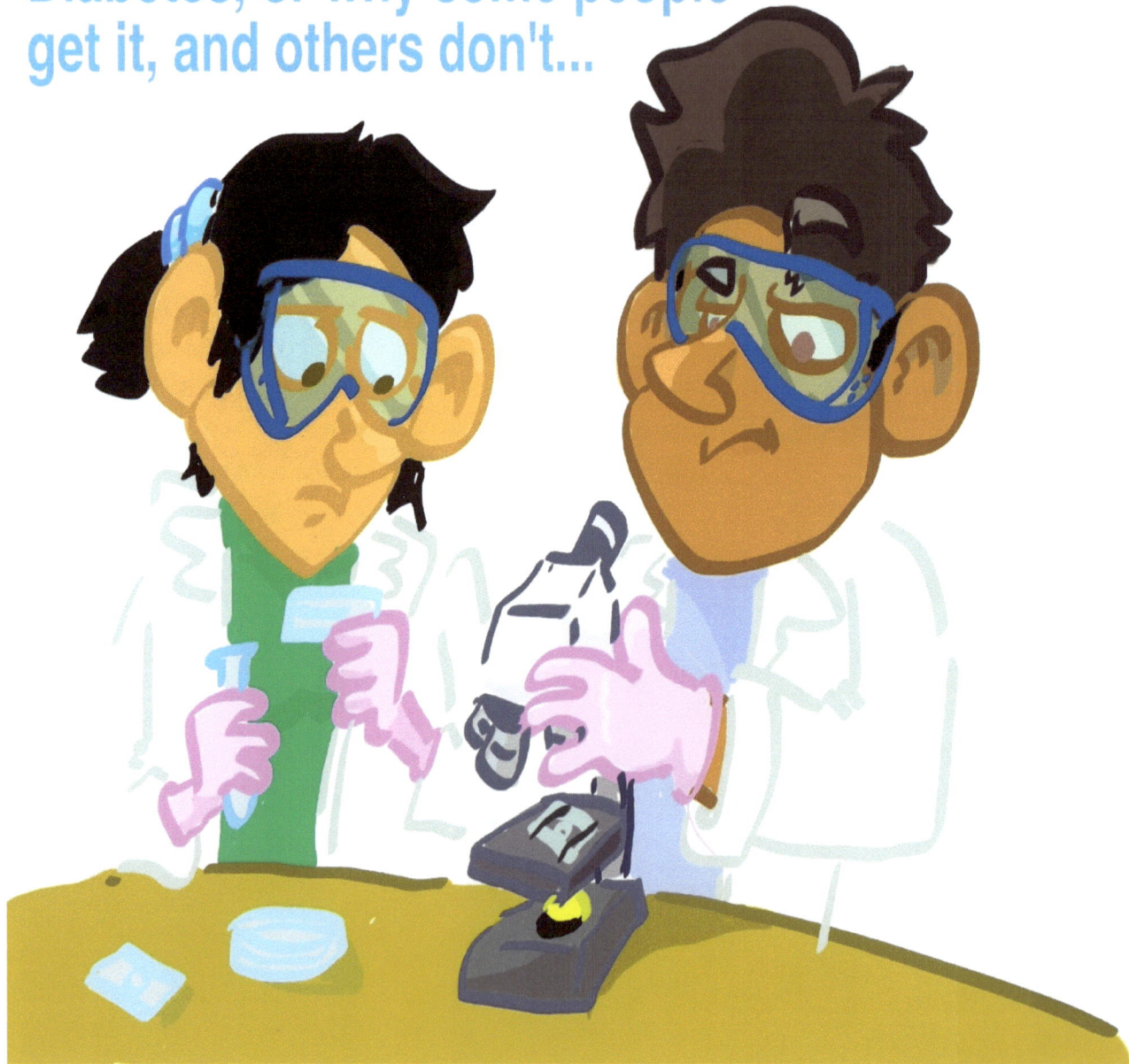
Scientists still aren't entirely sure what causes Type 1 Diabetes, or why some people get it, and others don't...

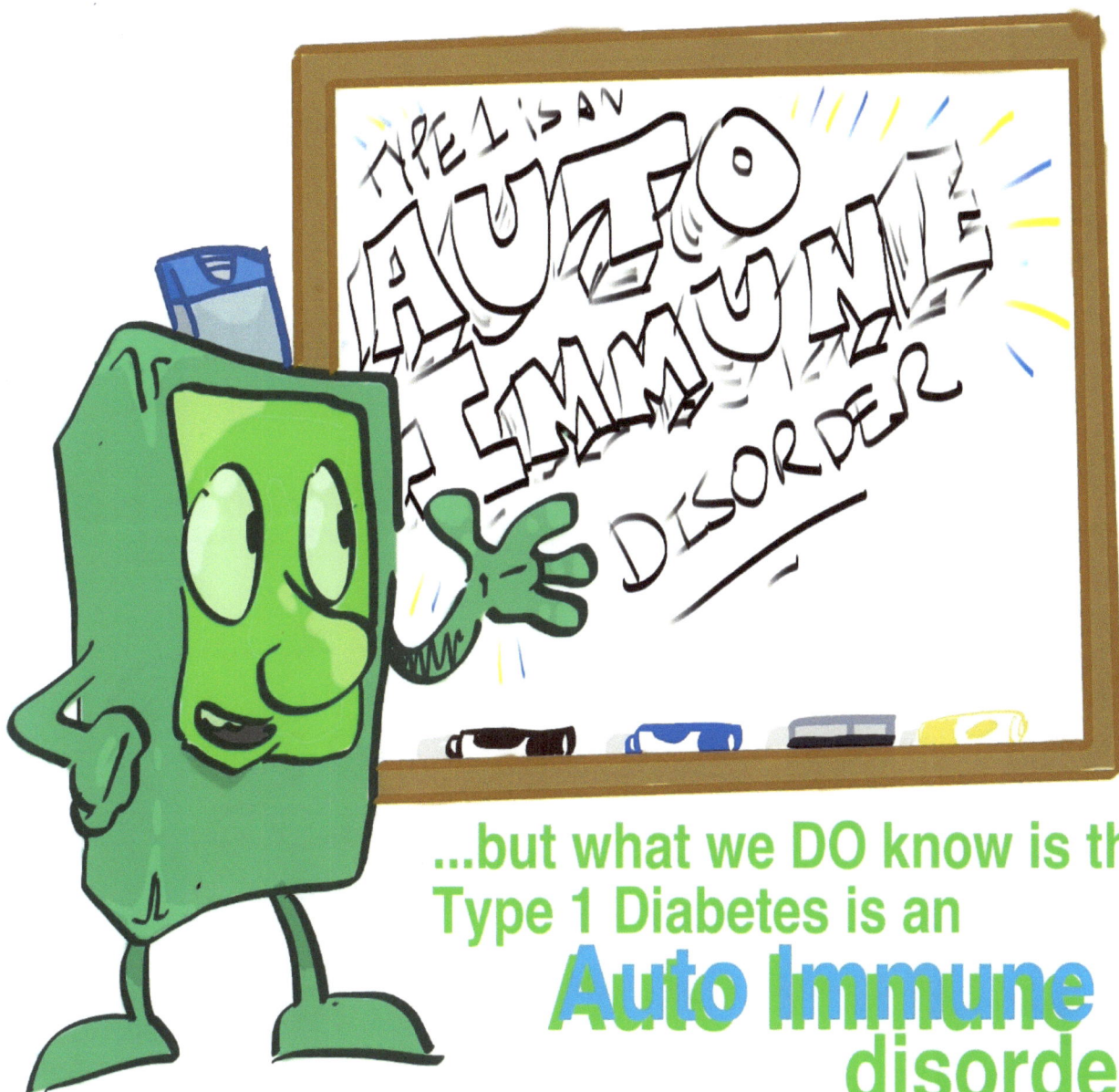

TYPE 1 IS AN AUTO IMMUNE DISORDER

...but what we DO know is that Type 1 Diabetes is an Auto Immune disorder...

The immune system protects your body from

harmful bacteria

and viruses.

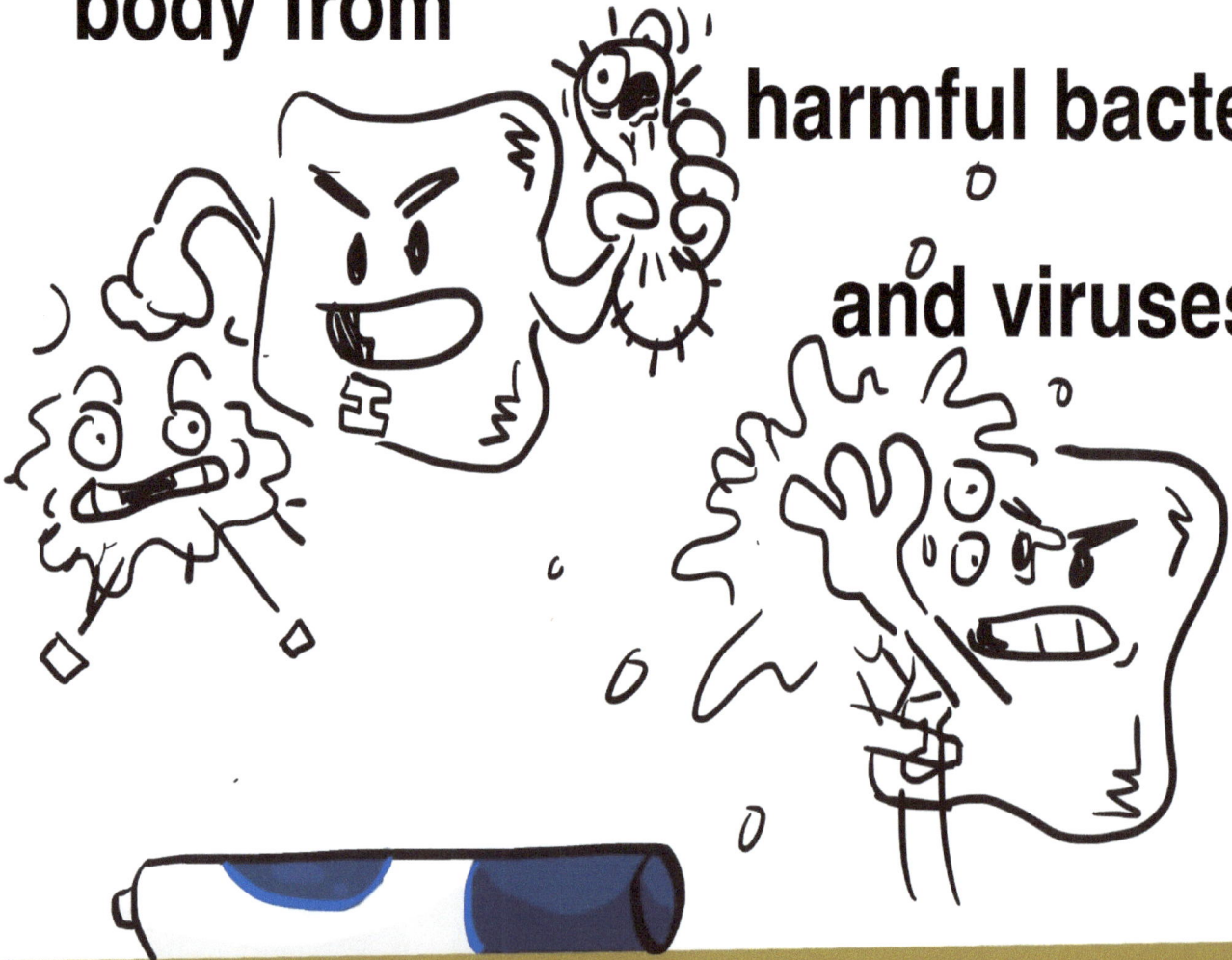

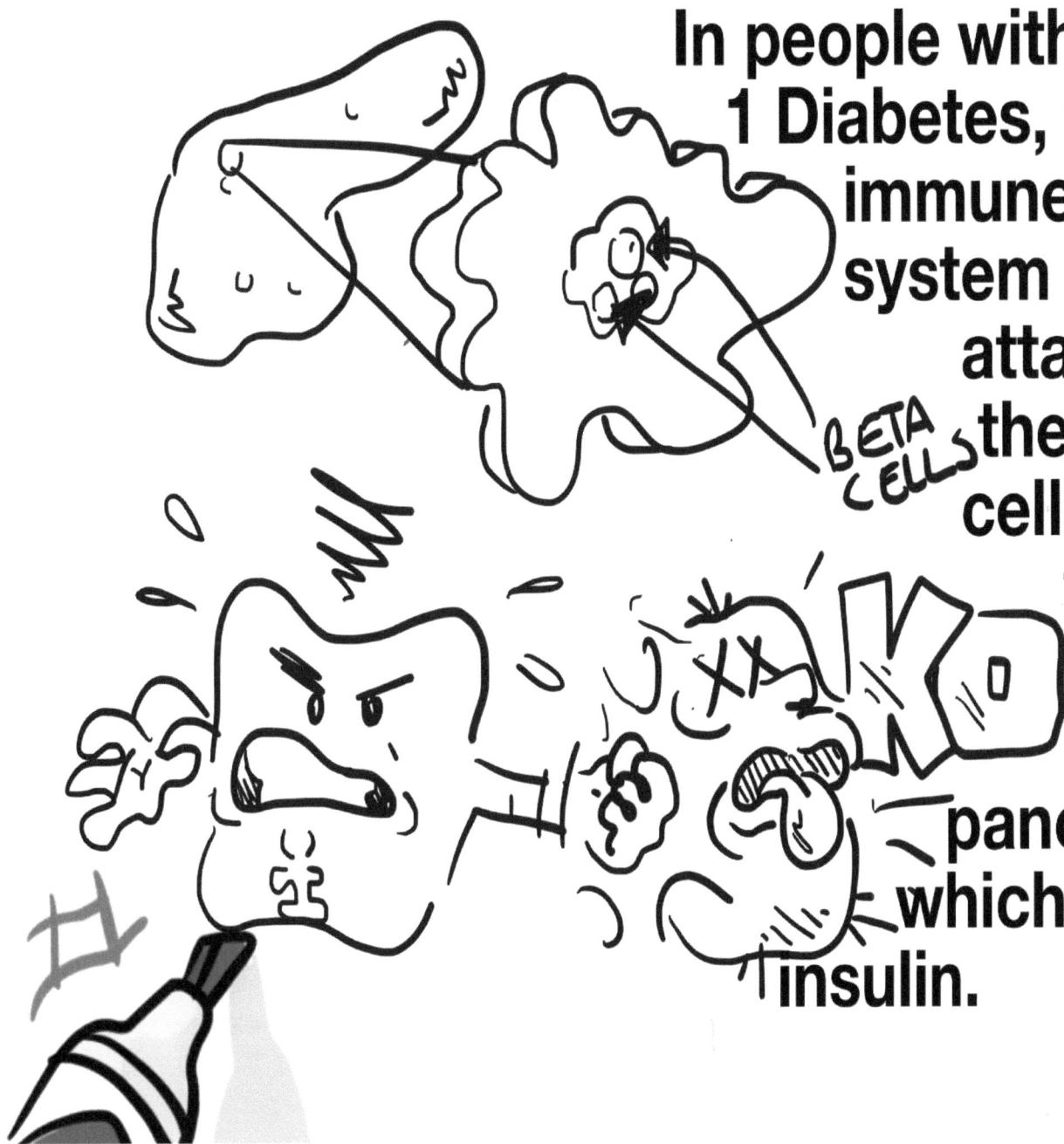

In people with Type 1 Diabetes, the immune system also attacks the beta cells in the pancreas which make insulin.

Fortunately, scientists have found that if the body stops attacking the beta cells, the remaining beta cells and beta cells that are transplanted into the body will be able to make insulin again! There are actually medicines that can cause this to happen.

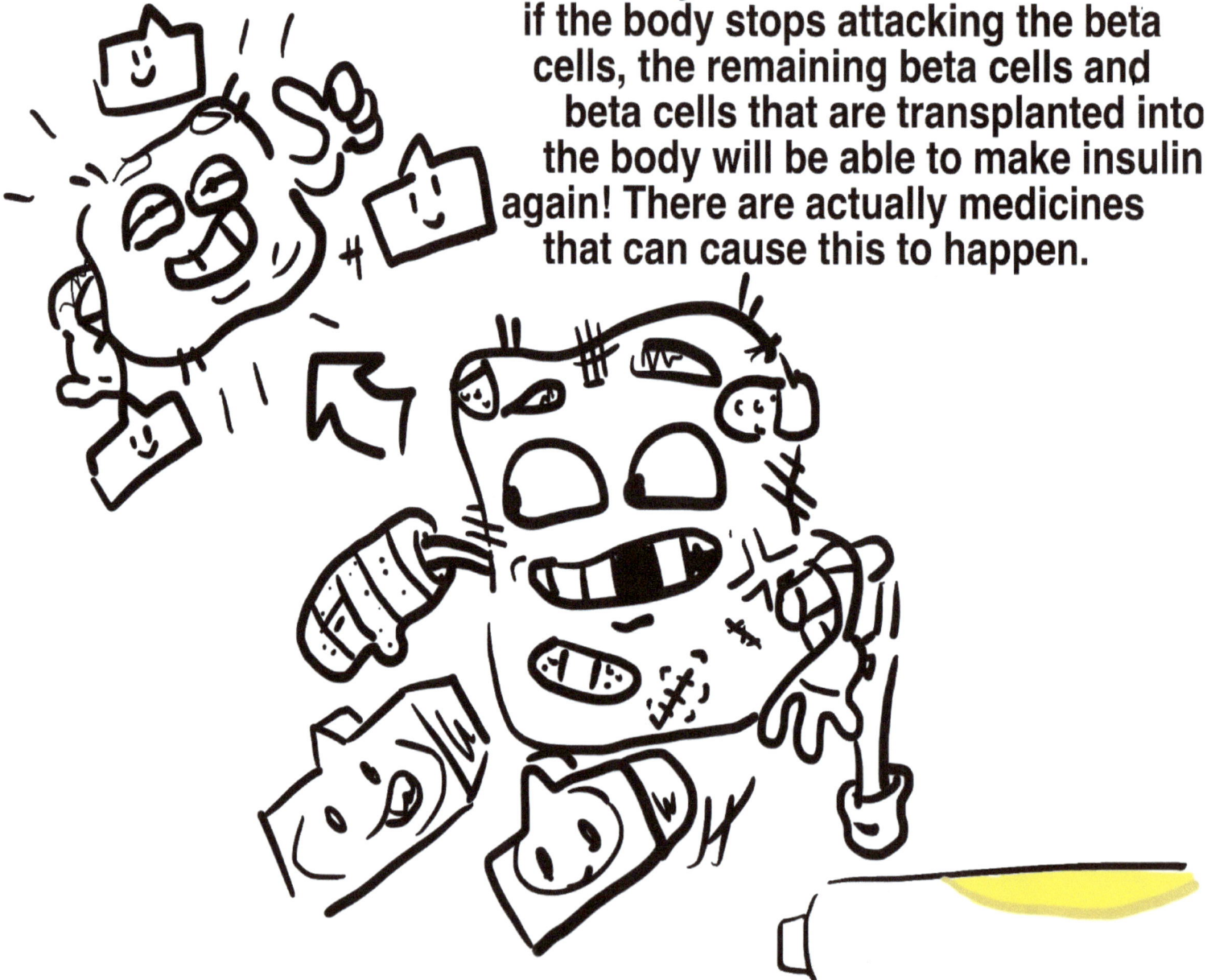

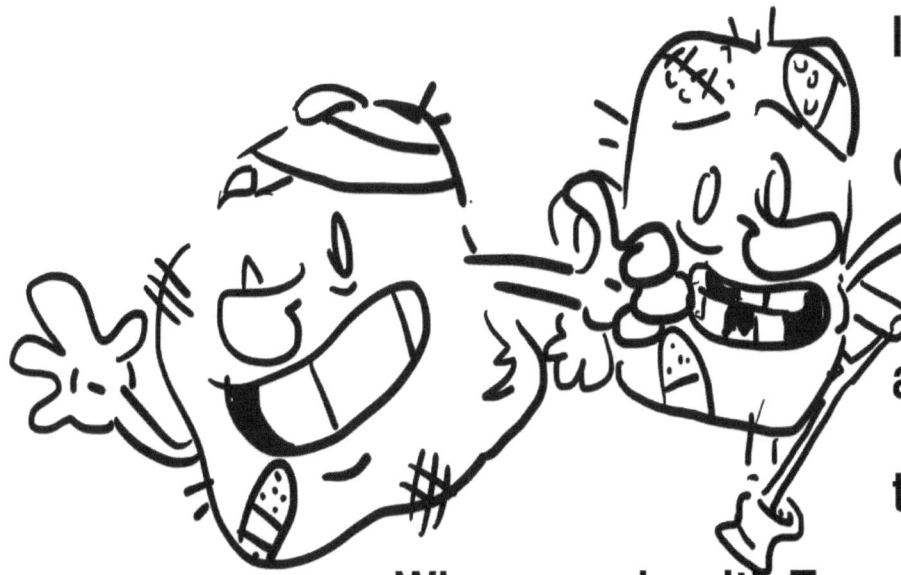

Immune suppressor drugs hold back the immune system. They interfere with the immune system's ability to function normally and attack things.

When people with Type 1 Diabetes take these drugs, it can help stop the immune system from attacking beta cells.

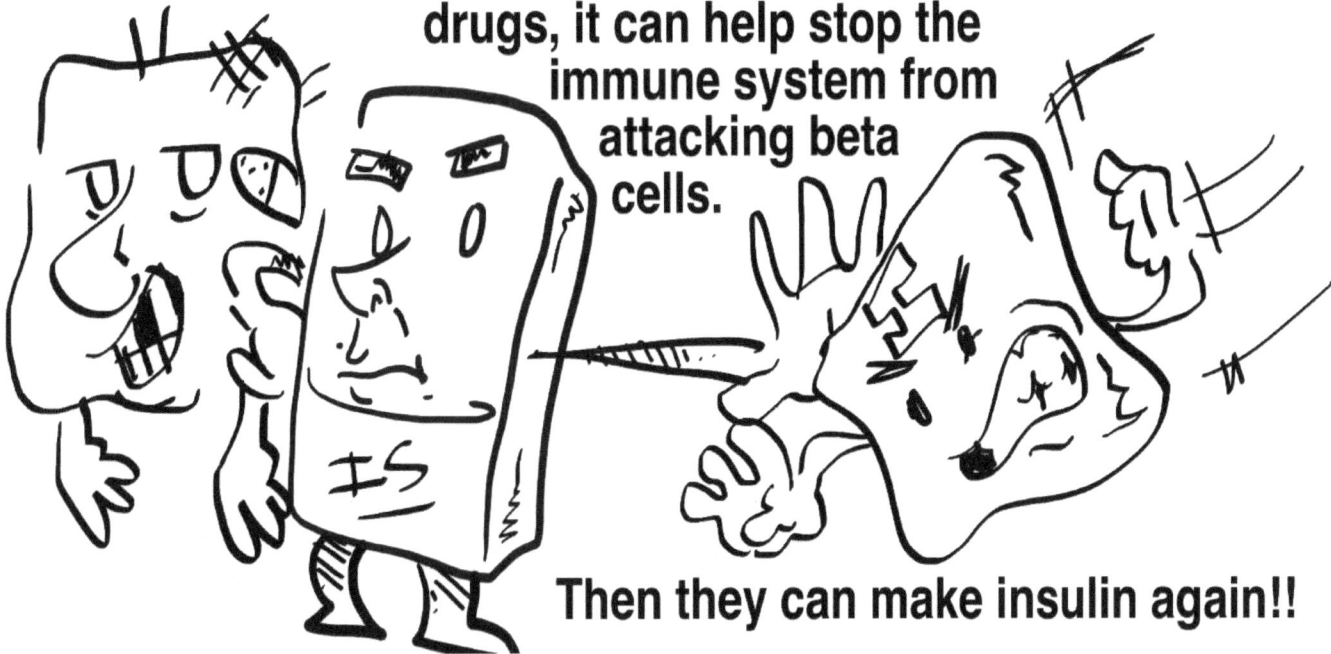

Then they can make insulin again!!

Sadly, these medicines don't just stop the immune system from attacking beta cells. They make it very difficult for it to attack anything.

This means the immune system has trouble attacking the bacteria, viruses and other bad germs that make you sick. So, people on these types of drugs can get very sick, and they can get sick very often. This can be much worse for your body than diabetes, so most diabetics use other treatments

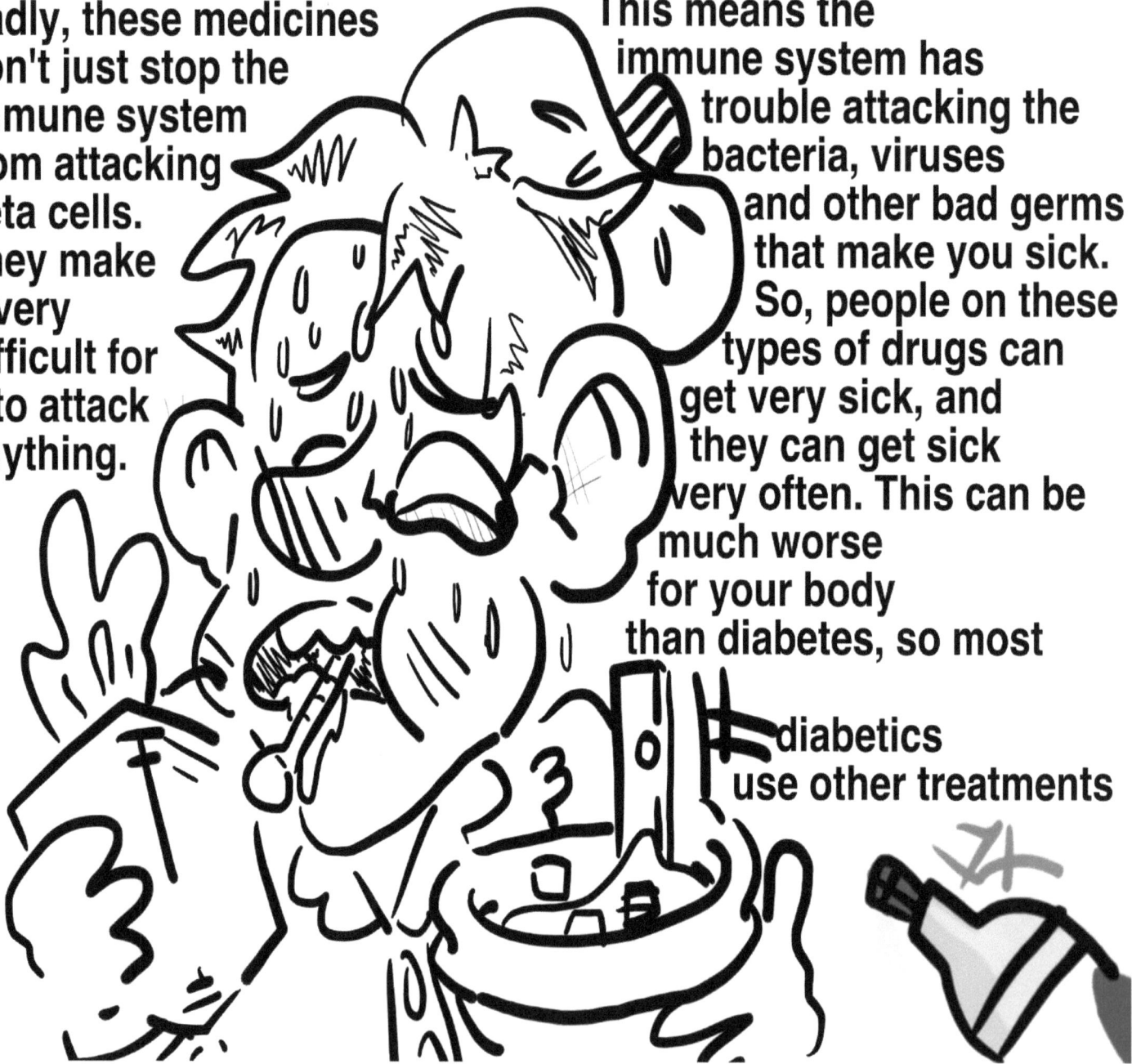

Fortunately, scientists have been able to make insulin that type 1 diabetics can take in place of the insulin that their pancreases can't make.

Now, people with diabetes live long happy, healthy lives!

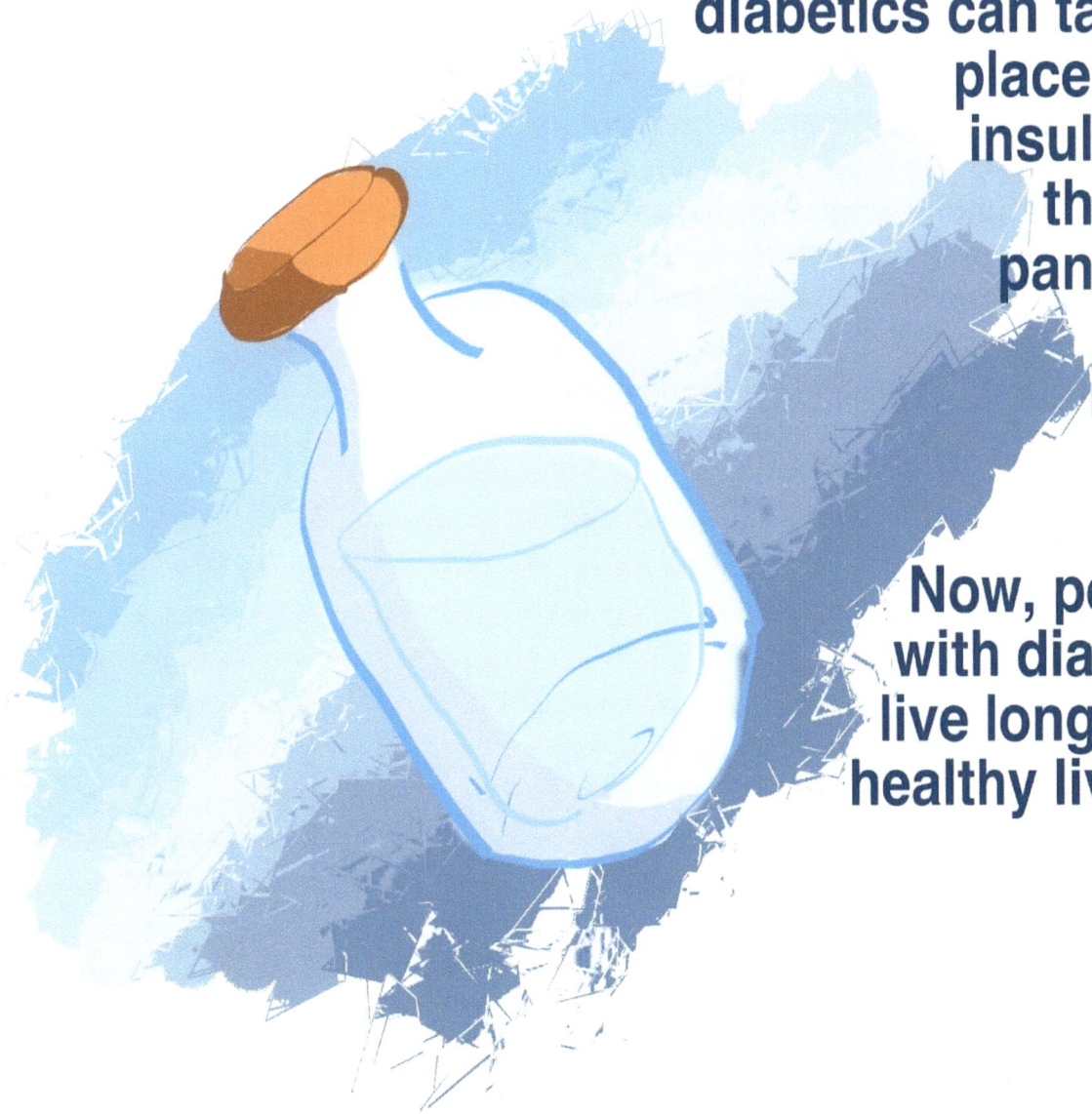

There are several ways diabetics can recieve their insulin doses.

Other diabetics use
insulin pumps
to get their insulin.

Some diabetics get insulin through insulin shots.

Insulin shots can come in the form of
insulin pens
or
syringes.

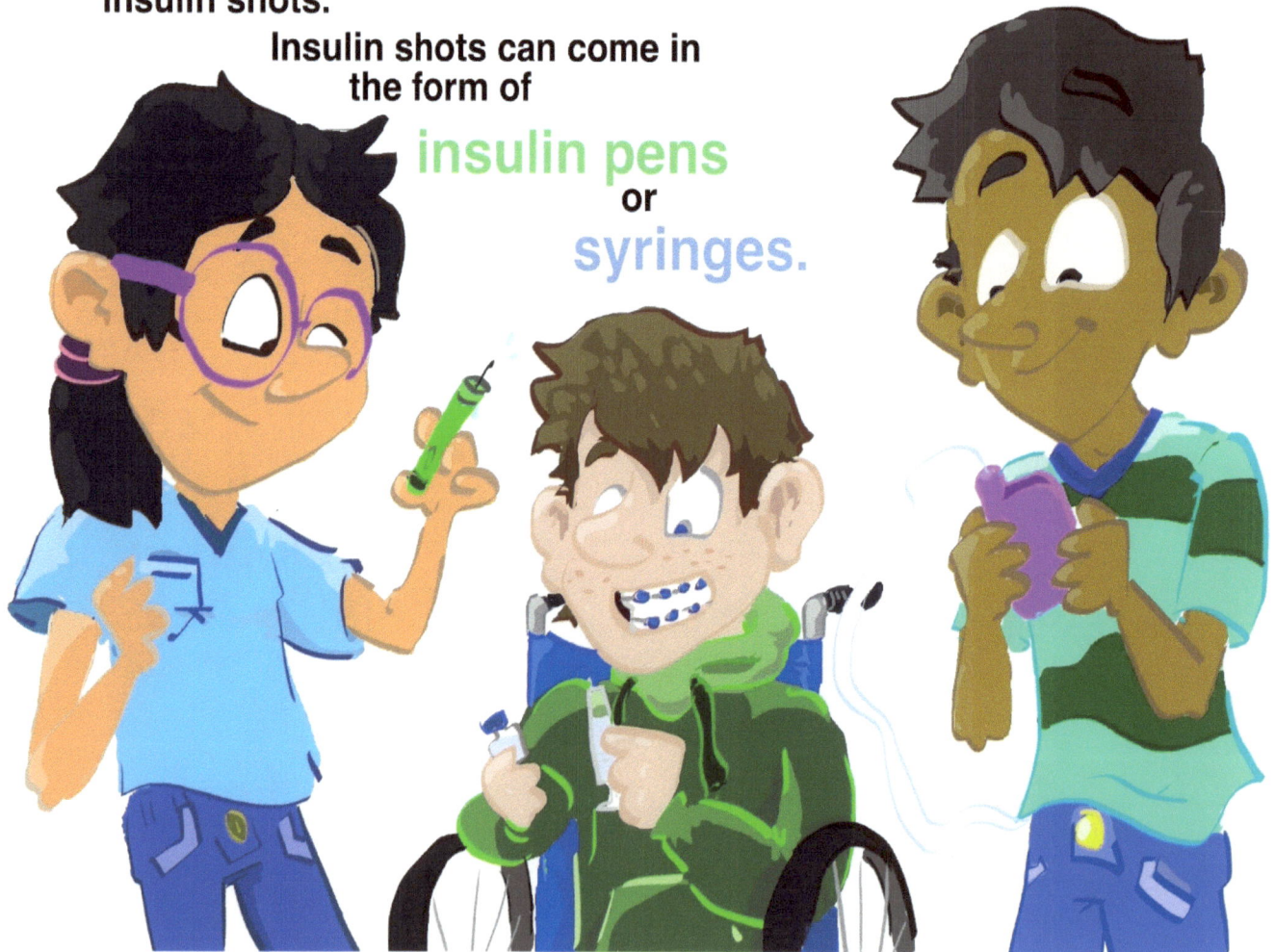

Insulin pens are re-usable, but the needles on the tops of pens need to be replaced after each use

Insulin pens use insulin from insulin cartriges, which you insert into the pen and replace when they expire or run out of insulin.

Insulin pens also usually include a dial which allows you to set the dose amount, and a button you press to deliver the insulin.

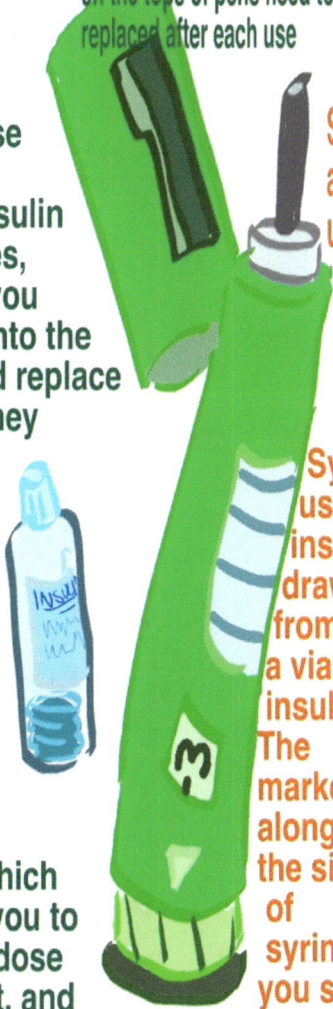

Syringes are not re-usable and a new syringe must be used for each insulin injection.

Syringes use insulin drawn from a vial of insulin. The markers along the sides of syringes help you set the correct insulin dose.

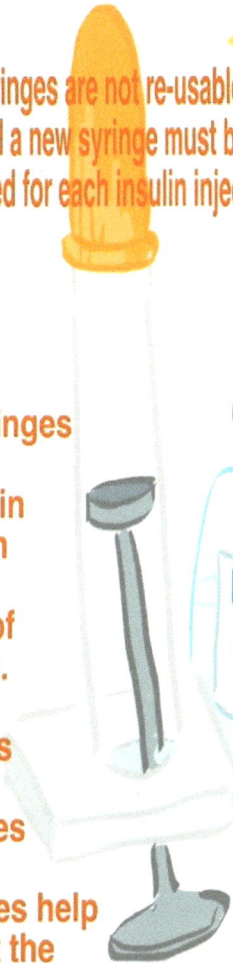

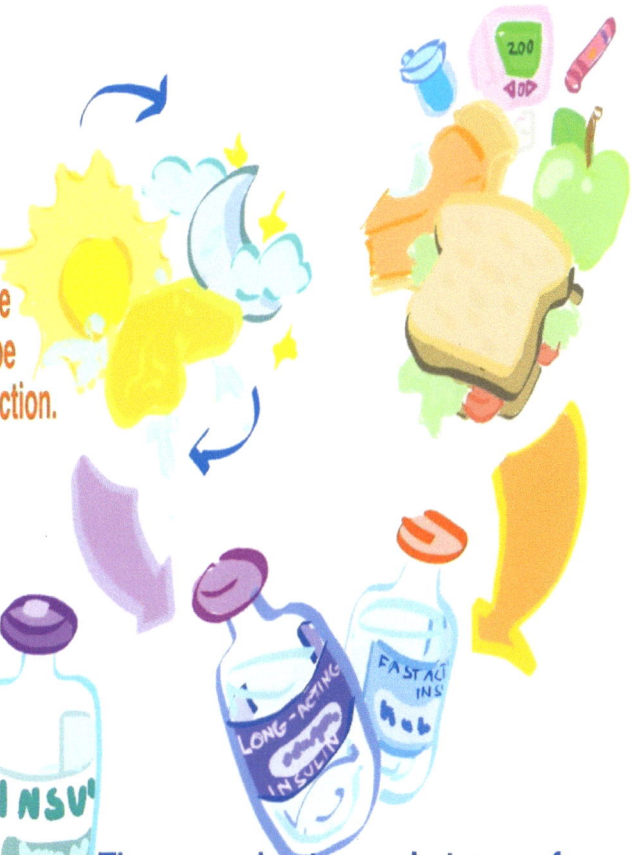

There are also two main types of insulin. Fast acting or short acting insulin is usually used to correct for high blood sugars or for carbs before or after eating. It behaves the most like natural, pancreas produced insulin. Long acting insulins usually work over 12 or 24 hours, and are designed to replace the extra insulin released by non-diabetic pancreases throughout the day.

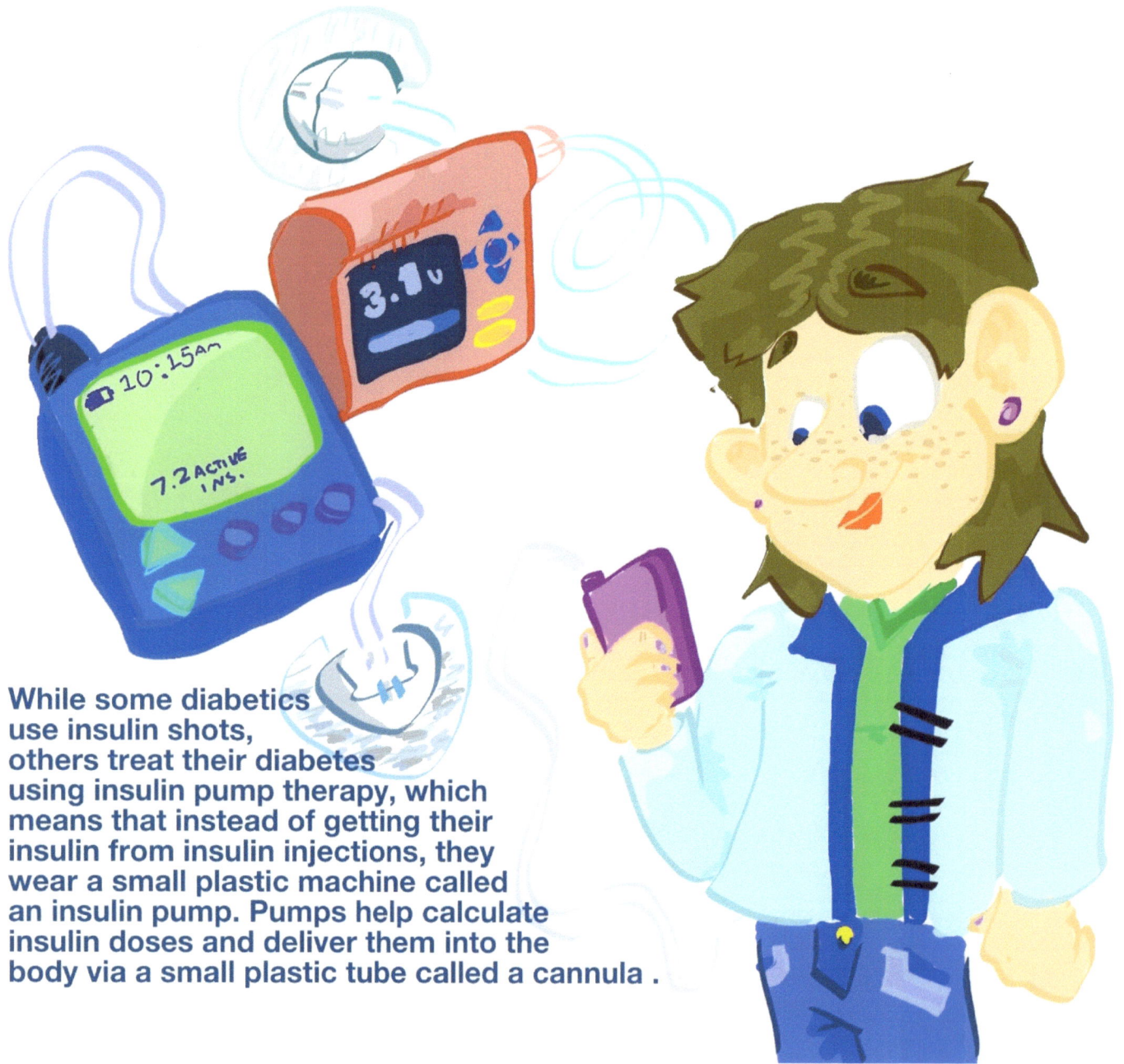

While some diabetics
use insulin shots,
others treat their diabetes
using insulin pump therapy, which
means that instead of getting their
insulin from insulin injections, they
wear a small plastic machine called
an insulin pump. Pumps help calculate
insulin doses and deliver them into the
body via a small plastic tube called a cannula .

Most pumps are water resistant (but not water proof), so they'll be ok if they're splashed or fall into something.
It's still not a good idea to take a shower or a bath or go swimming with one, unless the manufacturer and your doctor says you can.

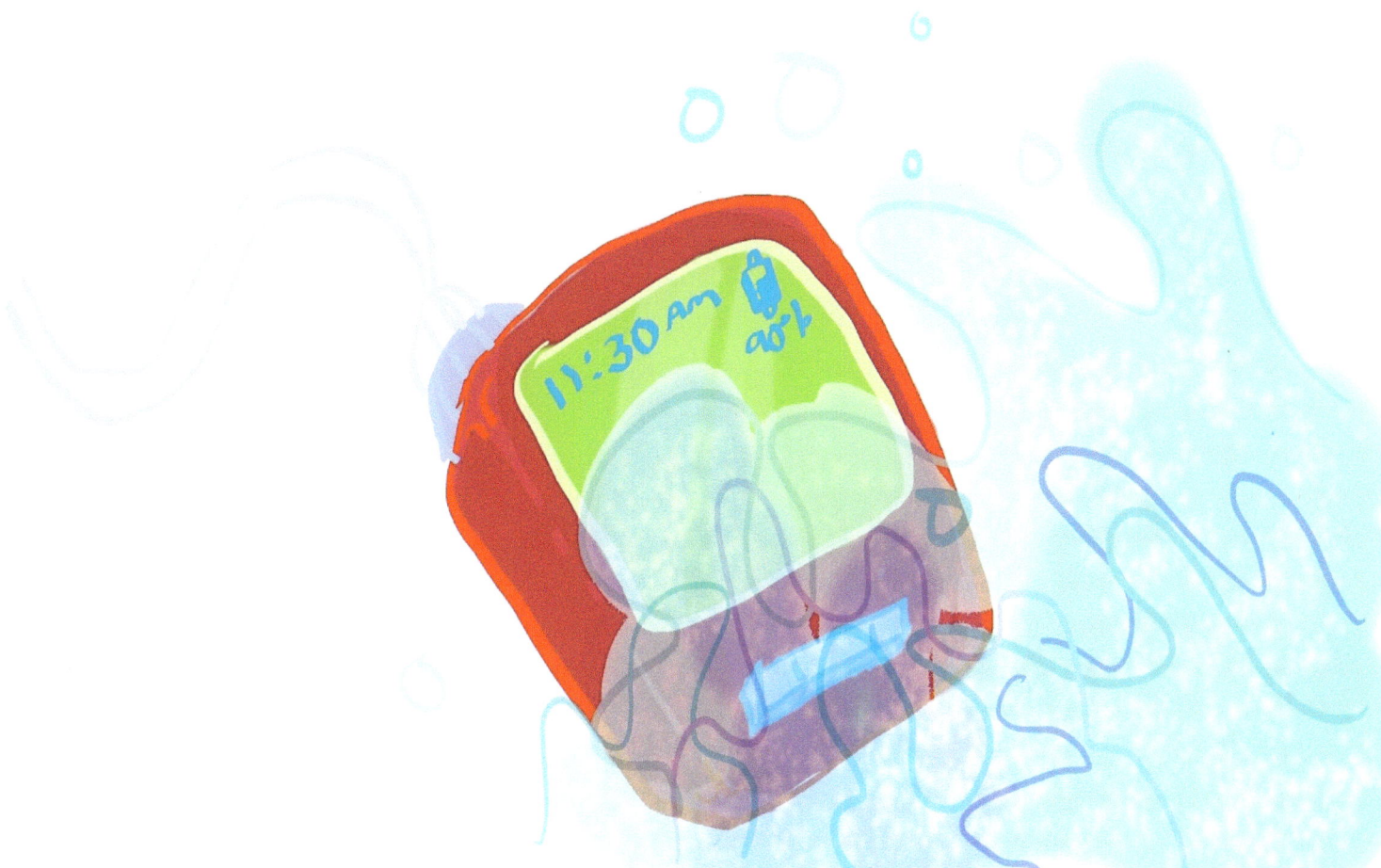

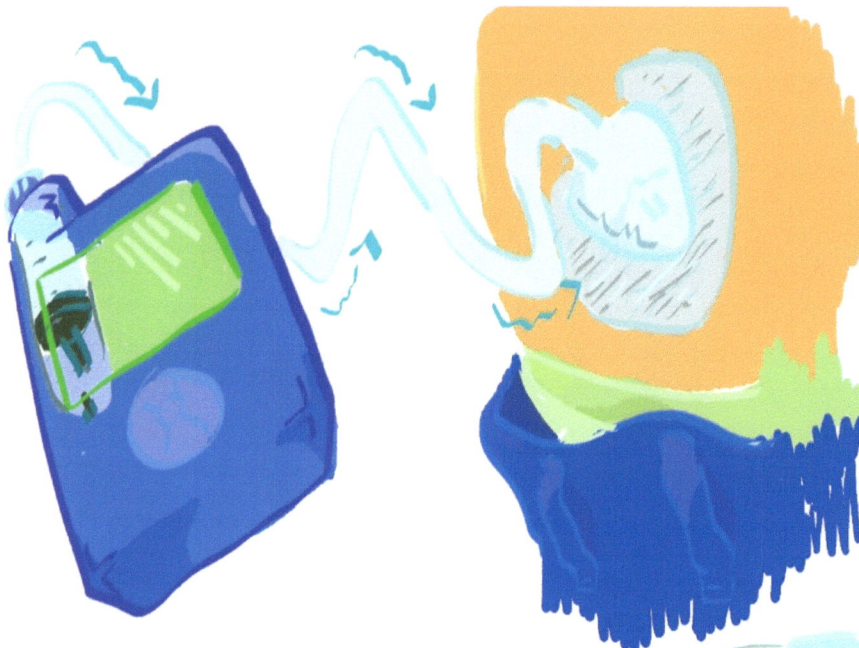

Insulin pumps deliver insulin by pushing insulin from a container inside the pump (known as a reservoir) through a thin, clear tube. The insulin travels through the tube into the infusion site--the plastic piece that connects the pump to the body--and into the cannula--the tiny plastic tube that extends from the skin--before entering the body. A common misconception is that the cannula is a needle. The cannula is not a needle. It is actually a very small plastic tube. Pump users use needles to insert cannulas into their bodies, but no needles stay in their bodies. The sites are designed so that the needles can be easily removed after the site has been inserted.

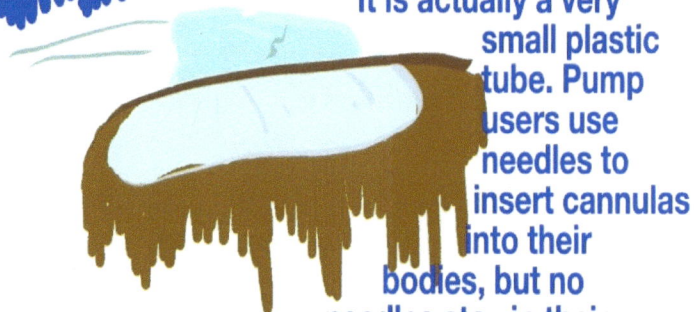

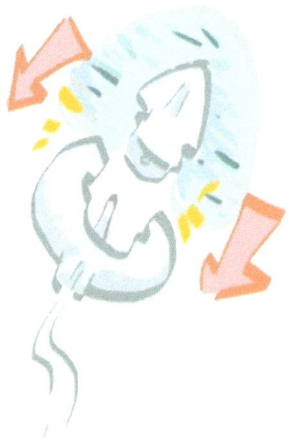

Luckily, insulin pump sites are designed to have the ability to disconnect from the pump and tubing temporarily, so people with pumps can disconnect from them to swim, shower, or take a bath. Some pump sites may come with a cap. The cap is usually shaped like the end of the pump's tubing so that it can click into the site while the pump's wearer swims, protecting the site. Ask your doctor about site caps and swimming while on insulin pump therapy, to know what's right for you and your pump.
Your doctor may also recommend that you take breaks from swimming to reconnect your pump if you're swimming or disconnected for a longer period of time.

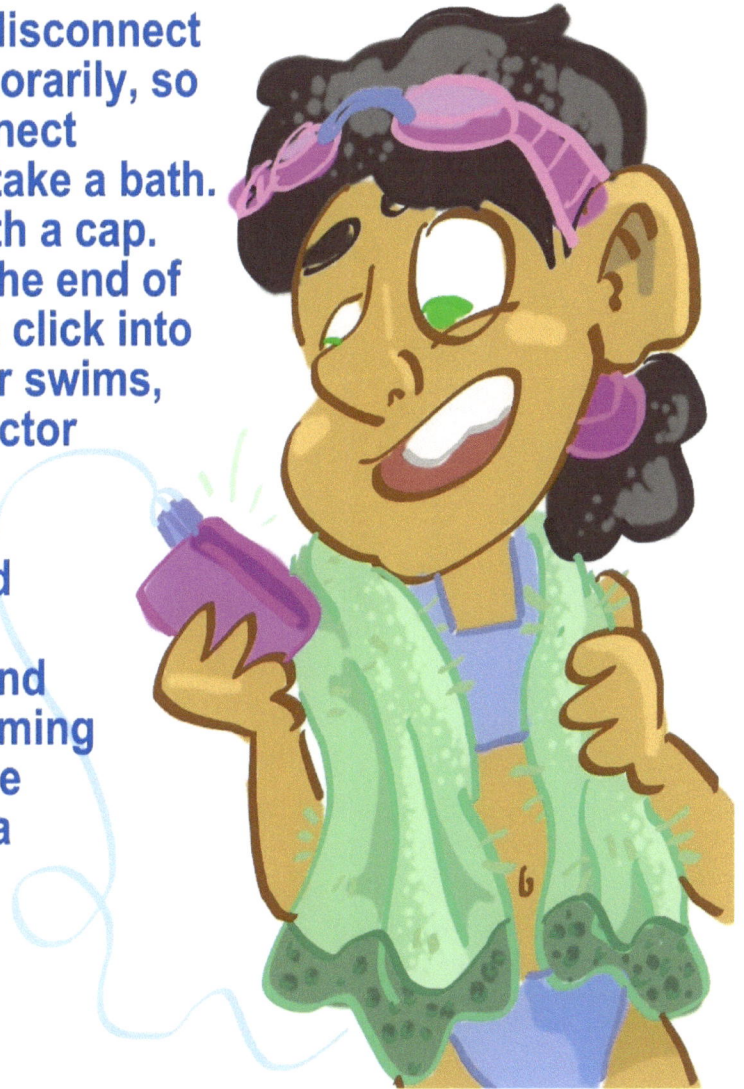

When should you give insulin?

Always follow your doctor's advice on giving insulin, but most people give insulin when they eat foods with

Carbohydrates, special molecules your body uses for energy that also raise the levels of glucose in your blood.

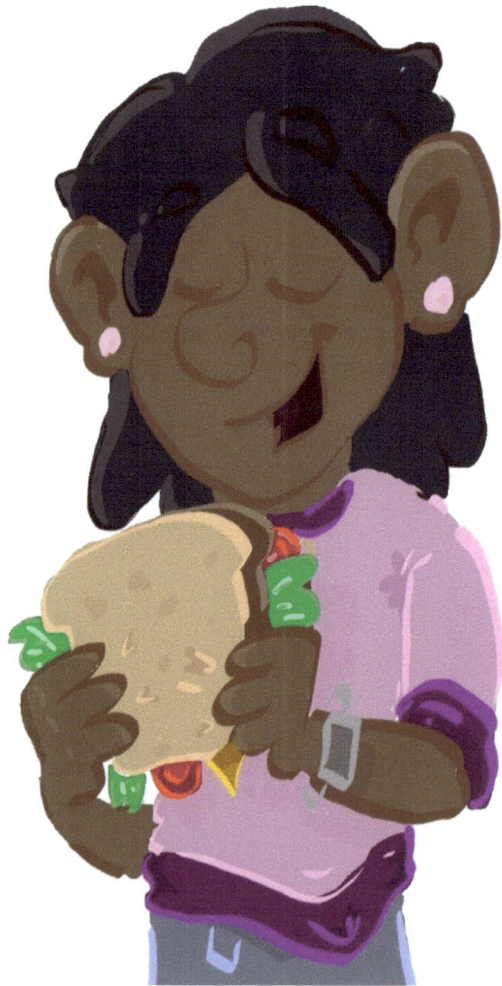

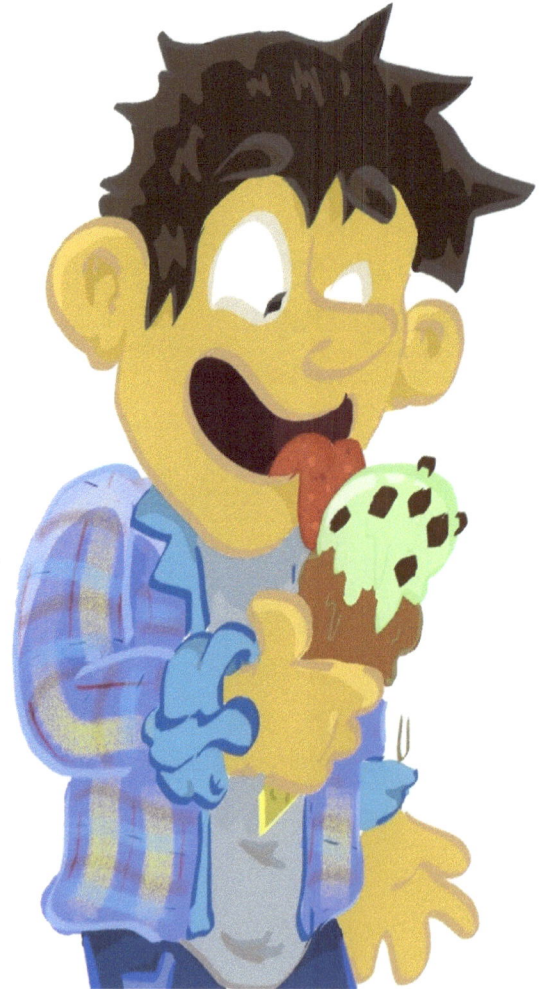

Blood sugar is the measure of the amount of glucose in your bloodstream, on its way to cells!

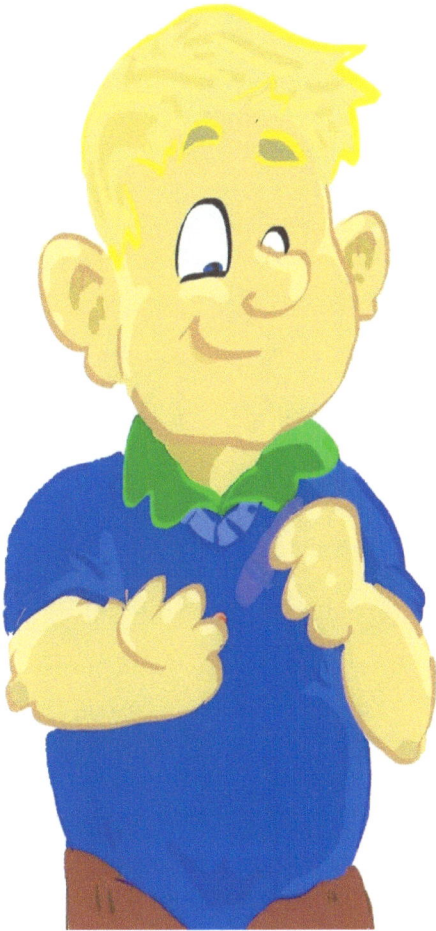

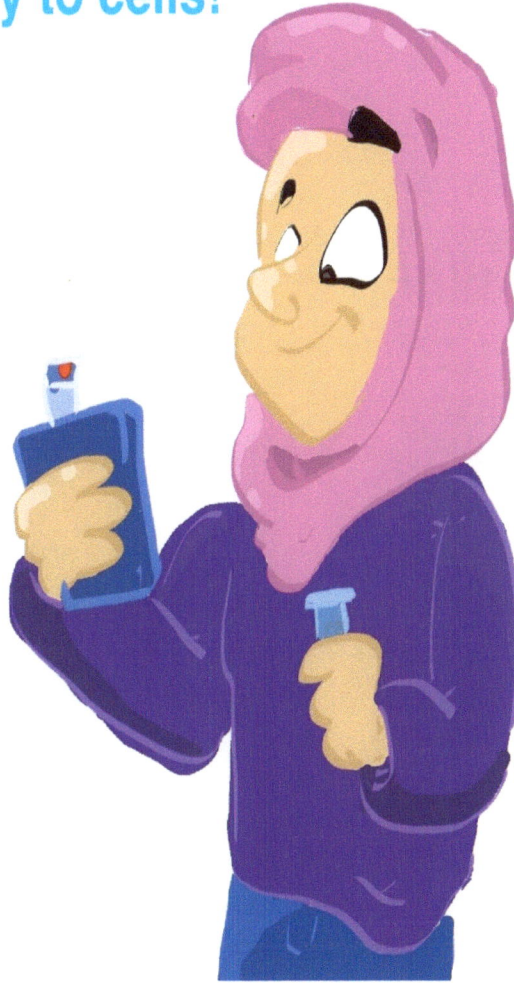

Blood Glucose Meters,

(which are also sometimes known as blood sugar meters, blood sugar testers, or testers)

measure blood sugar by using a tiny drop of blood from your finger tip. Most meters measure in mg/dl, which is short for milligrams (1/1000th of a gram) of glucose per deciliter (1/10th of a liter) of blood.

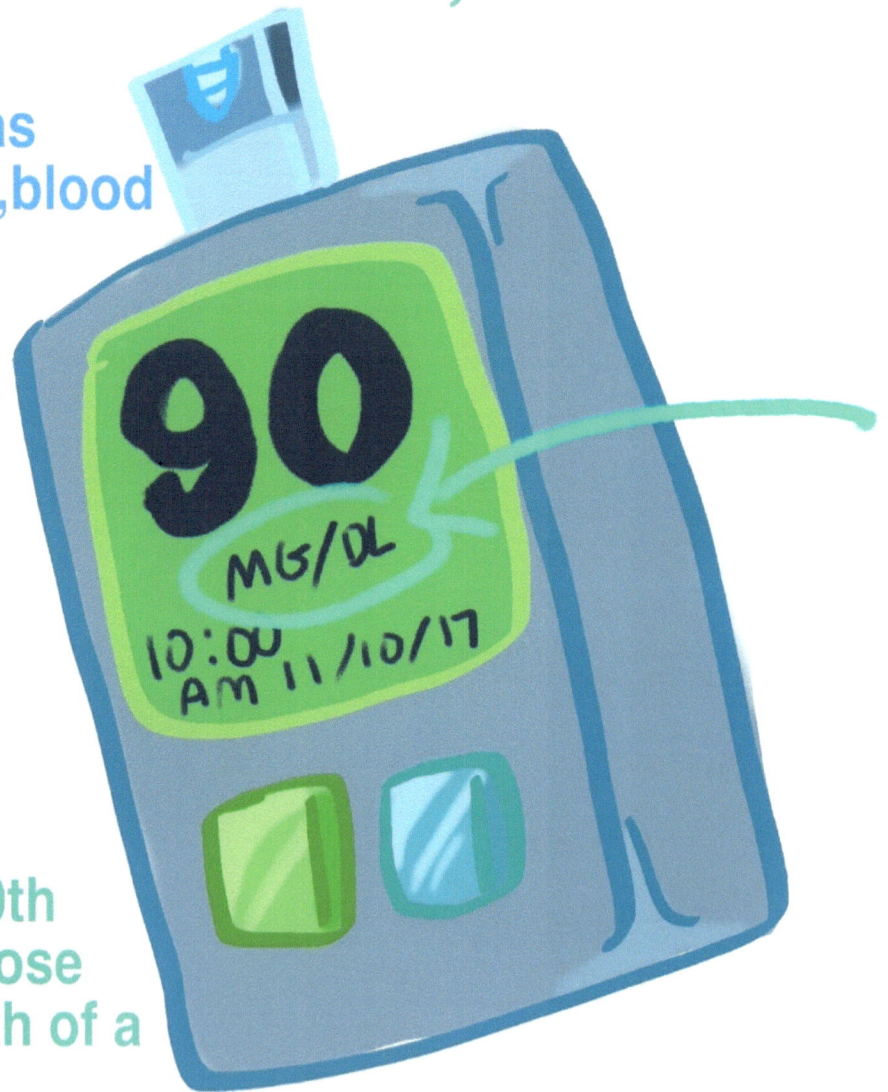

90
MG/DL
10:00 AM 11/10/17

Meters use tiny metal and plastic rectangular strips called test strips. The test strips fit into a slot in the meter and have a small area where you can place a tiny drop of blood you get from your fingertip using a device called a lancet. Lancets don't hurt much (it's just a tiny prick)--but they do take some getting used to. The blood drawn by the lancet that you put on the strip helps the meter tell you what your blood sugar is!

It's important to monitor your blood sugar closely with the help of your meter so that it doesn't go too high or low which will make you feel sick.

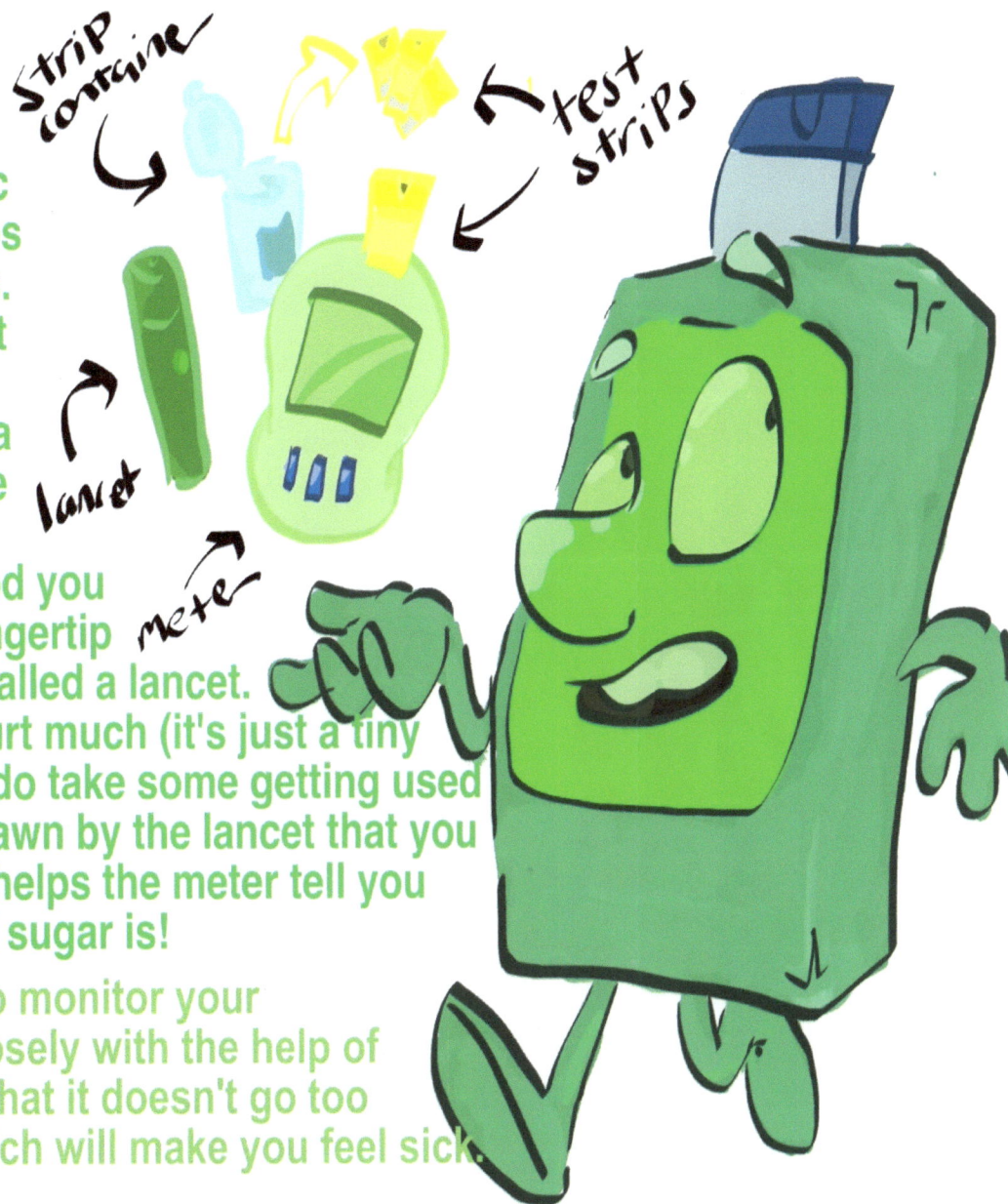

strip container

test strips

lancet

meter

Lots of things can affect your blood sugar. Stress, exercise, changes to your daily routine, and even growing can impact your blood sugar, so it's important to closely follow your doctor's advice on how to care for it!

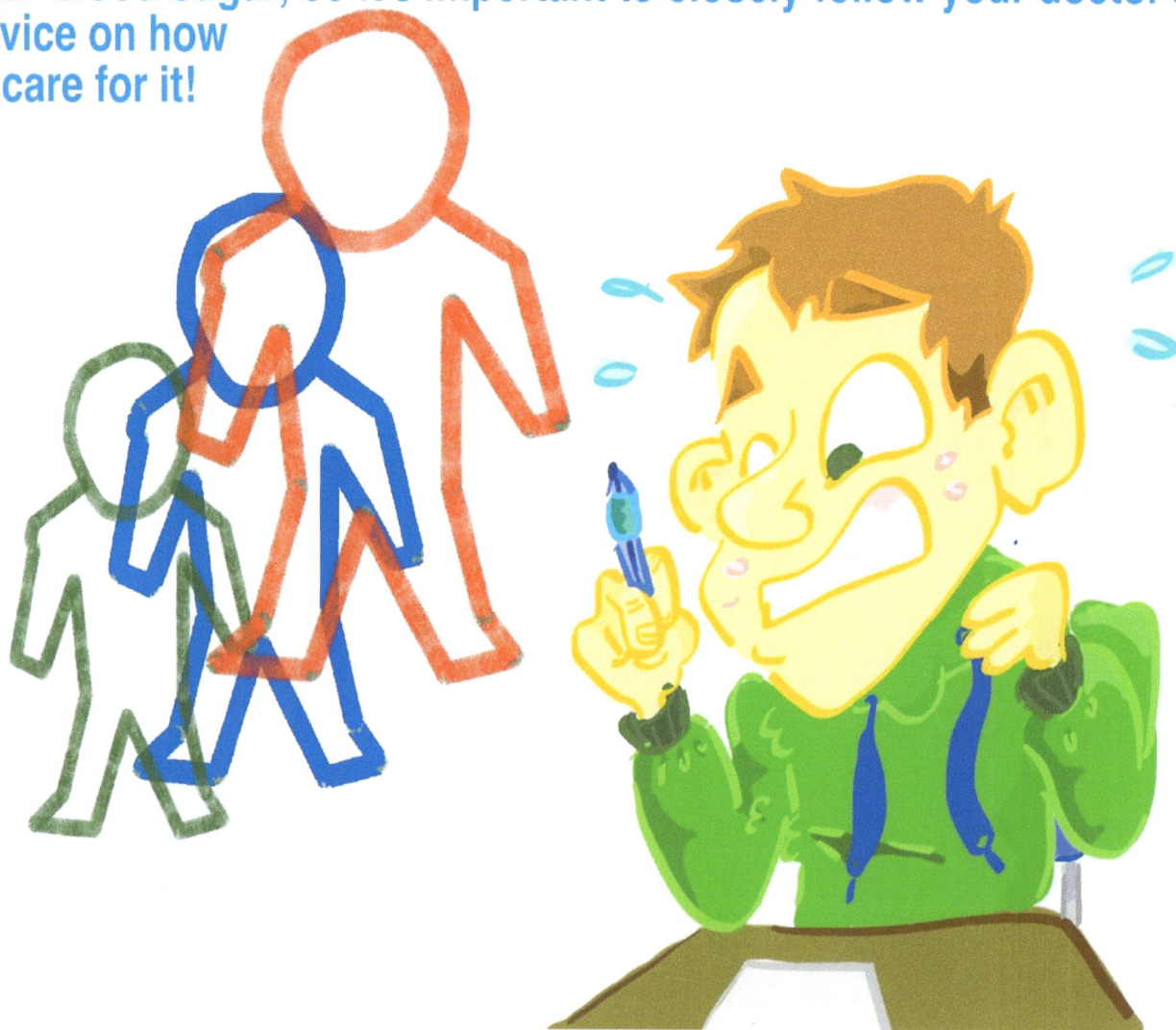

Being sick can also mess with your blood sugar, so you should pay extra attention to it if you're not feeling well. It can also make you more likely to develop diabetic ketones, which can be harmful and make you feel even more sick.

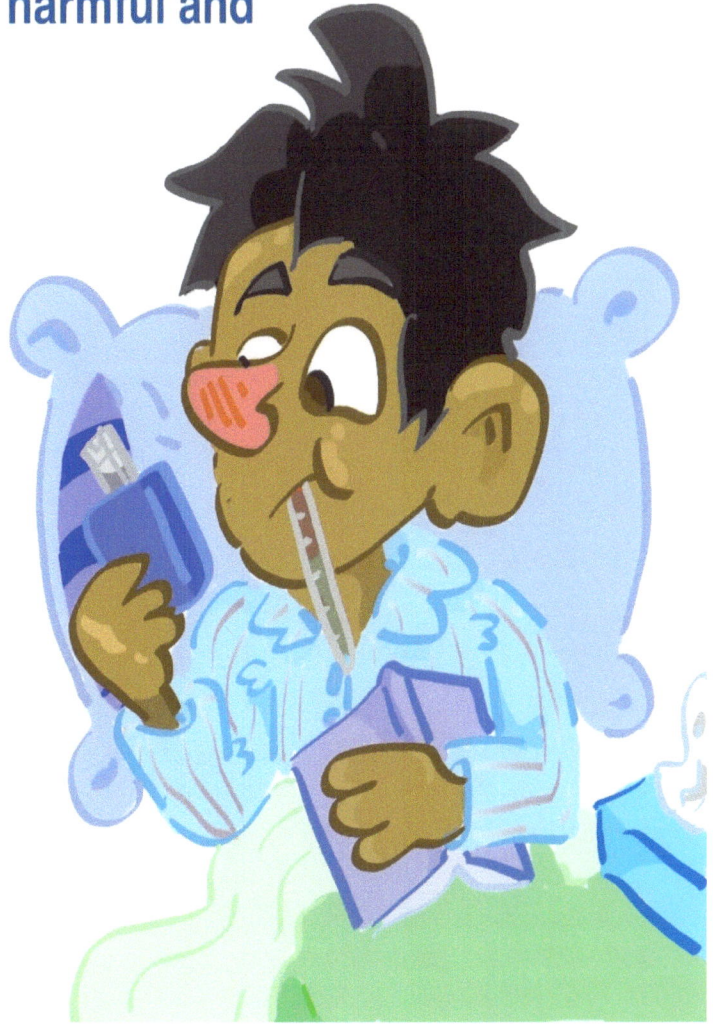

Ketones

are harmful acids
released by your
body. They can
show up if
you aren't
getting
enough insulin,
or when you're sick.
Ketones can make you
nauseous, dizzy, or have a "fruity"
or "metallic" taste in your mouth.
Ketones are part of why most diabetics
feel very icky when they are first diagnosed.

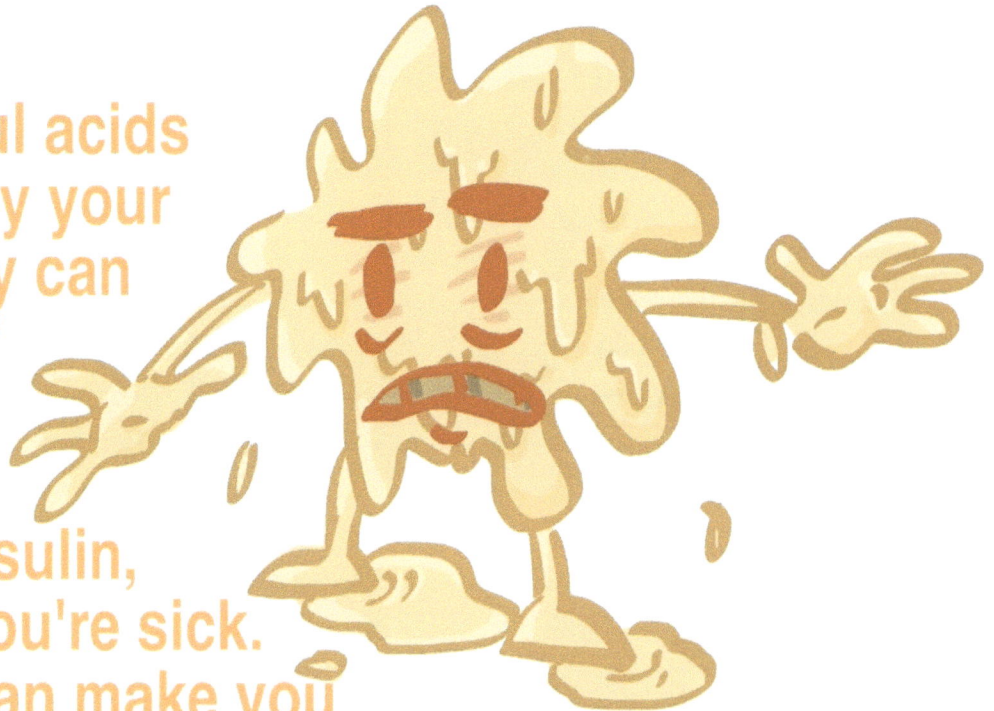

The liver is in charge of making ketones and sending them out into your body. Ketones evolved to help the body and cells stay fueled so they can do their jobs even when cells aren't taking in glucose they need for energy. The ketones help by breaking down fats to be used as energy.

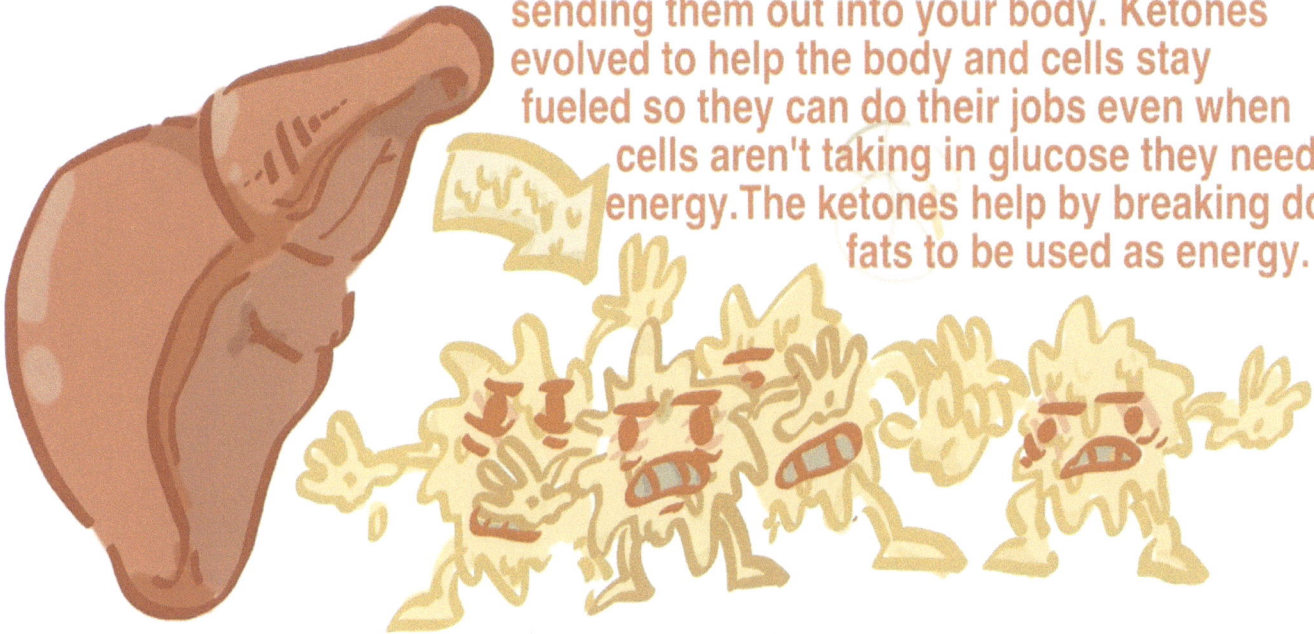

This helps the cells survive and do their jobs until glucose is available to be used as energy!

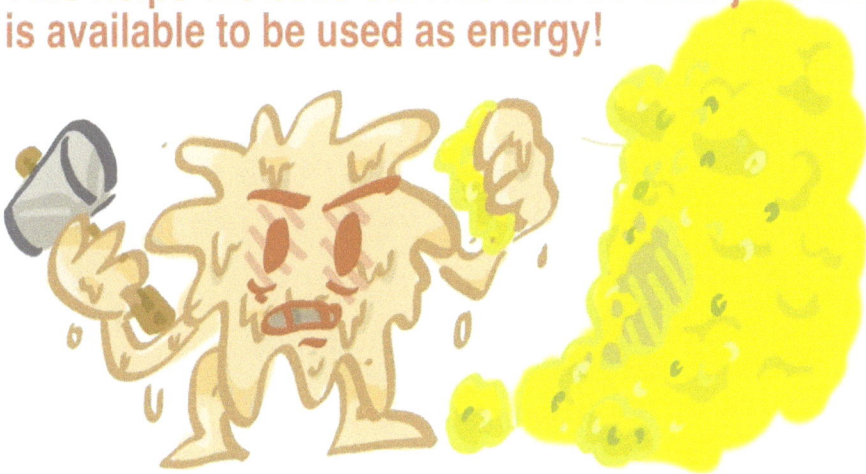

But because ketones can make you sick, and because they can also hurt important body parts, they're only used when your body thinks they're needed.

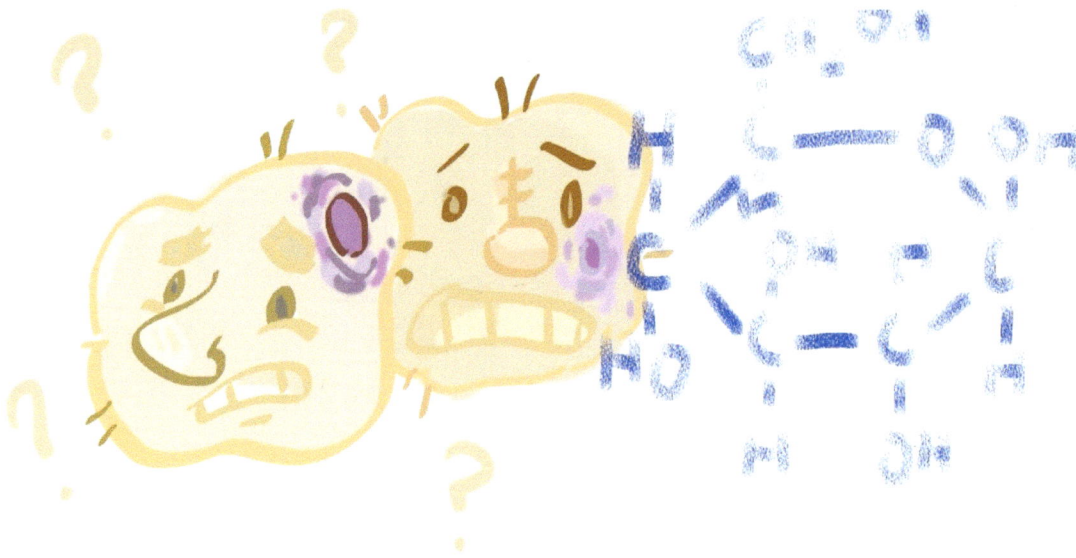

In Type 1 Diabetics, however, the problem isn't that their bodies don't have glucose. The problem is that the cells can't take in the glucose that is there because there is no insulin to tell them to.

The liver doesn't know this, however. It releases ketones to help the cells get energy since the body assumes the reason the cells aren't taking in glucose is because there is no glucose in the blood at all.

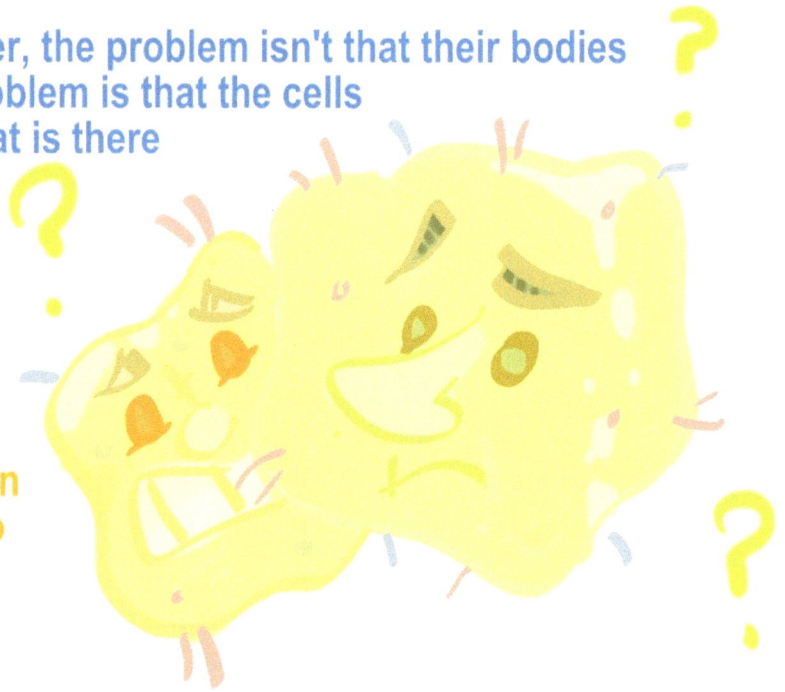

Because they are so harmful, the body will flush out ketones by making you thirsty so you drink lots of water. This makes you have to go to the bathroom, and the ketones are washed out of your body when you pee.

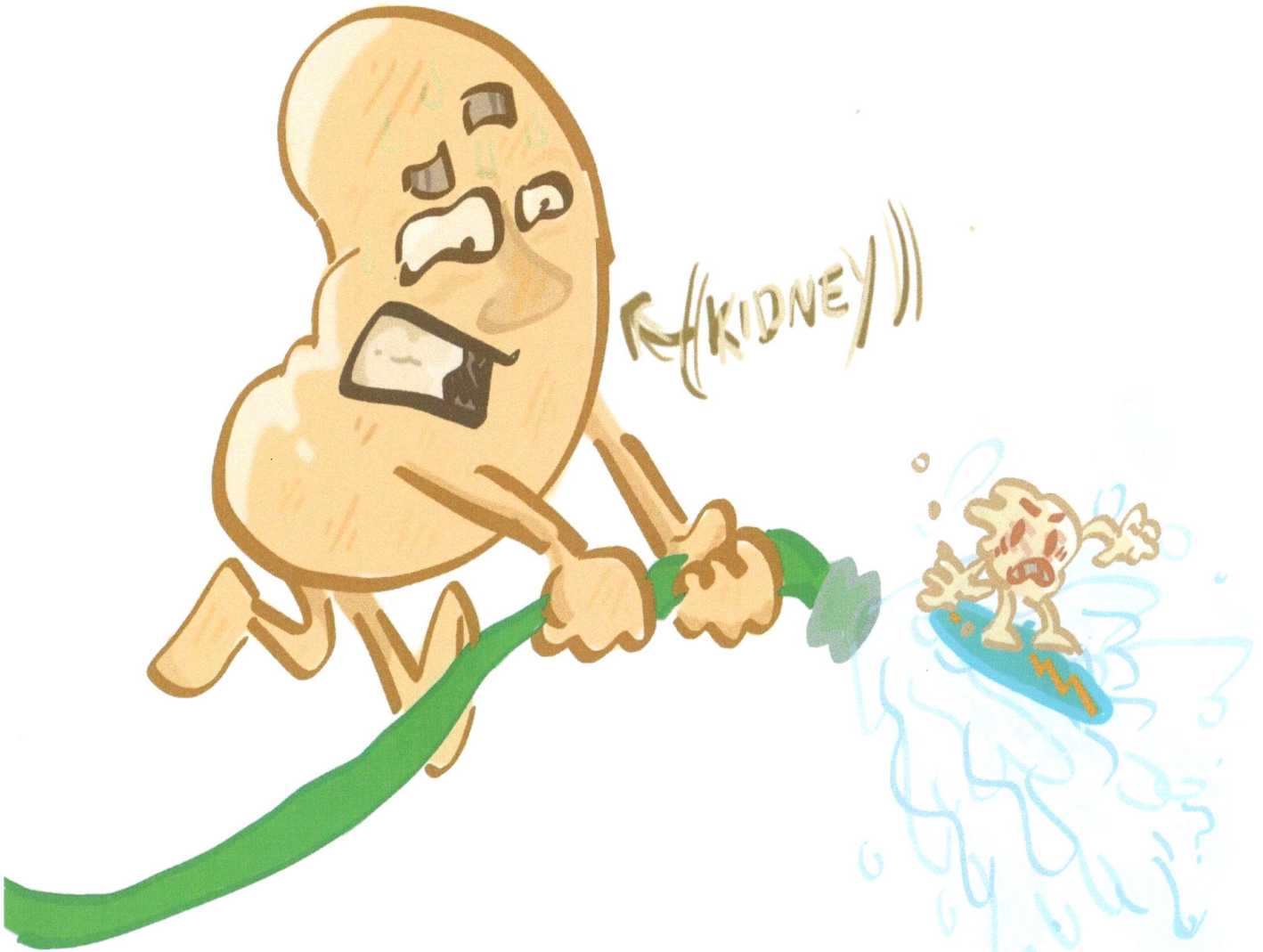

Ketone strips and meters exist that can help tell if there are ketones in your body. Ketone meters work like blood glucose meters and look for ketones in your blood.

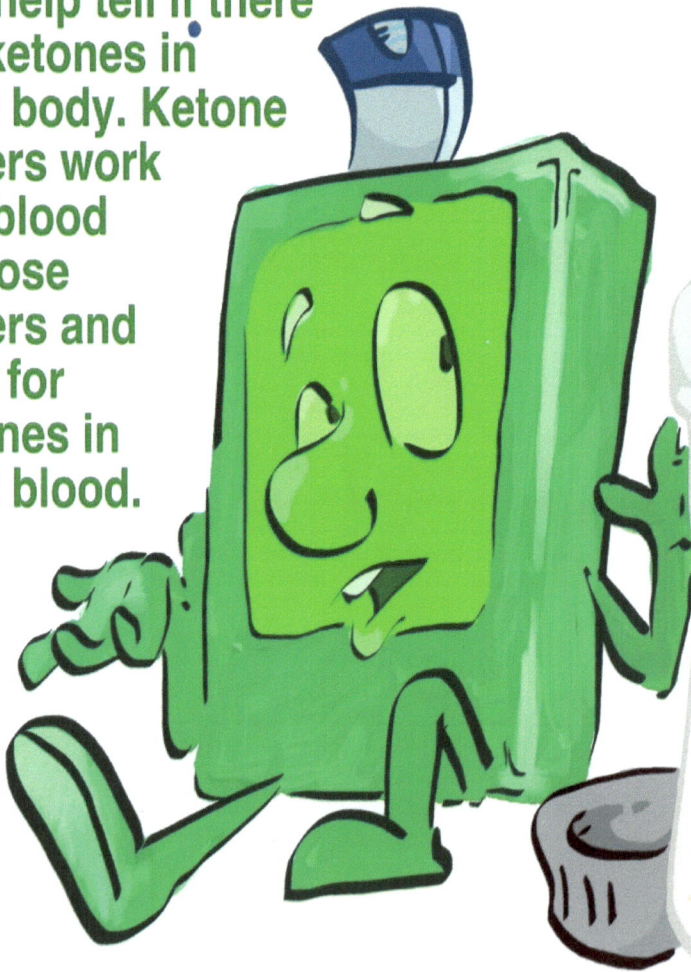

Ketone strips, like these, measure ketone levels in your pee. They can do this because the body tries to flush out the harmful ketones by sending them away with pee.

If you detect ketones, it's very important to follow your doctor's advice on how to get rid of them, and to drink water!

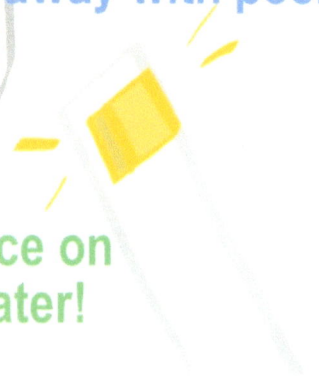

Hyperglycemia

is another name for high blood sugar. It can make you feel tired or thirsty and it can happen if you don't get enough insulin, eat a lot of carbs, or before your insulin kicks in and starts working!

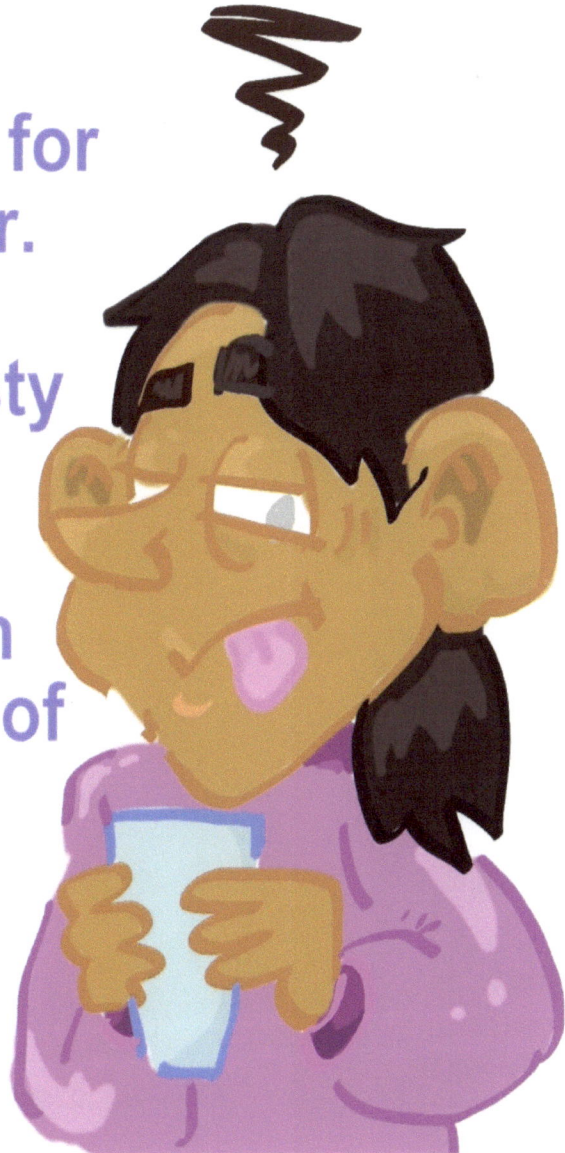

Hypoglycemia

is another name for low blood sugar. It can make you feel dizzy or weak.

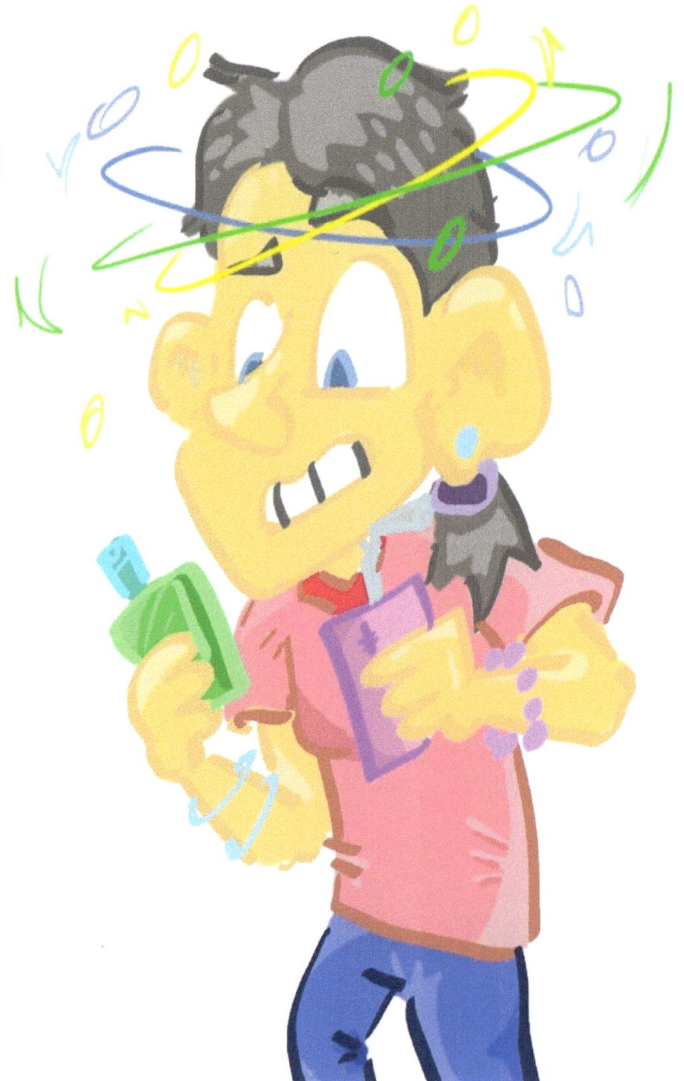

You can get low blood sugar for a variety of reasons. These include exercise, stress, and giving too much insulin.

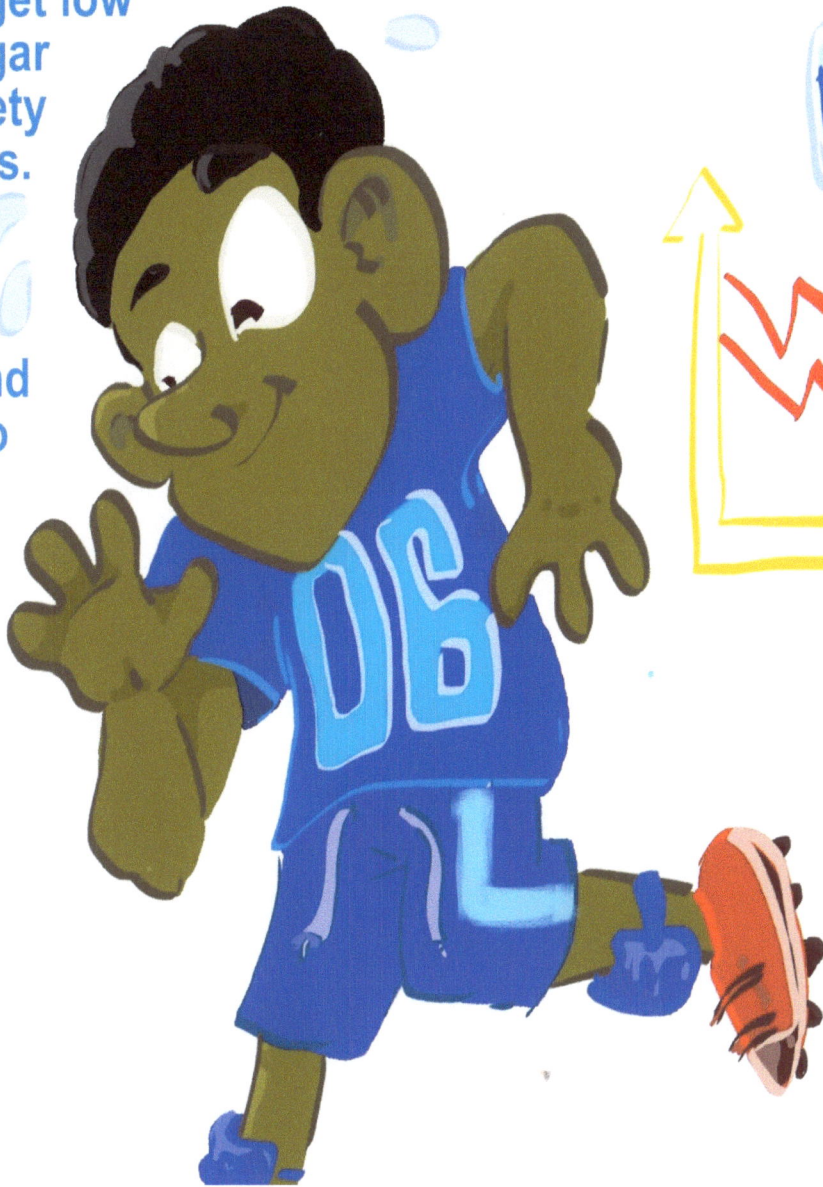

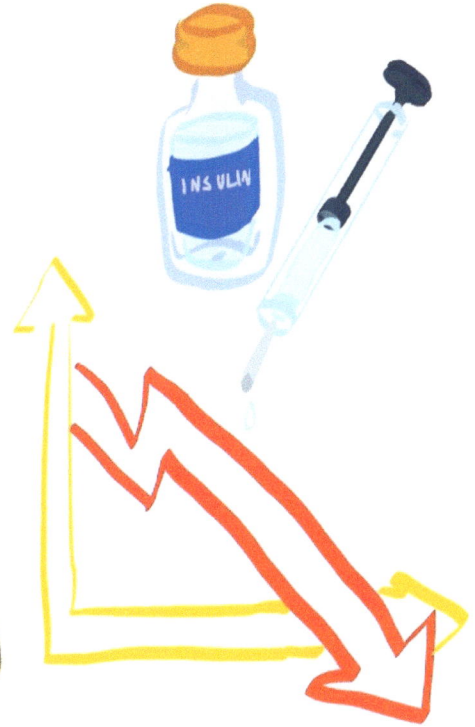

If your blood sugar goes low, it's important to eat or drink something so that it goes up. Glucose tablets and gels exist that are specially made to raise blood sugars, but you can also use juice, candy, fruit, or a variety of other sugary snacks.

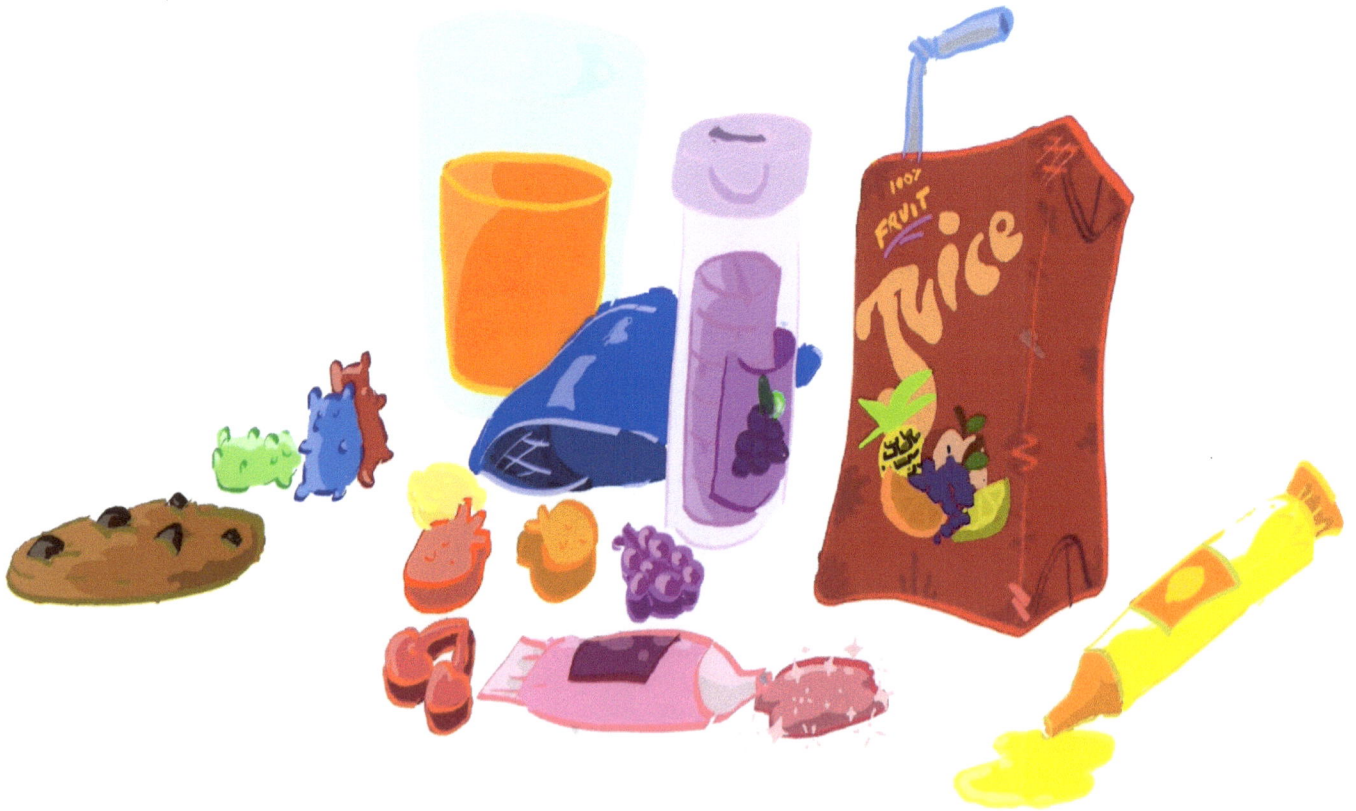

Although it's hard to deal with Type 1, or with any type of diabetes, Type 1 diabetics who take care of their diabetes live lives as long and healthy as those without diabetes. Never let diabetes stop you in life. Diabetics have achieved their dreams by becoming doctors, authors, buisnesspeople successful musicians, olympic atheletes and everything in between by using their tallents, passions, and the strength and resilience that comes from dealing with Type 1.

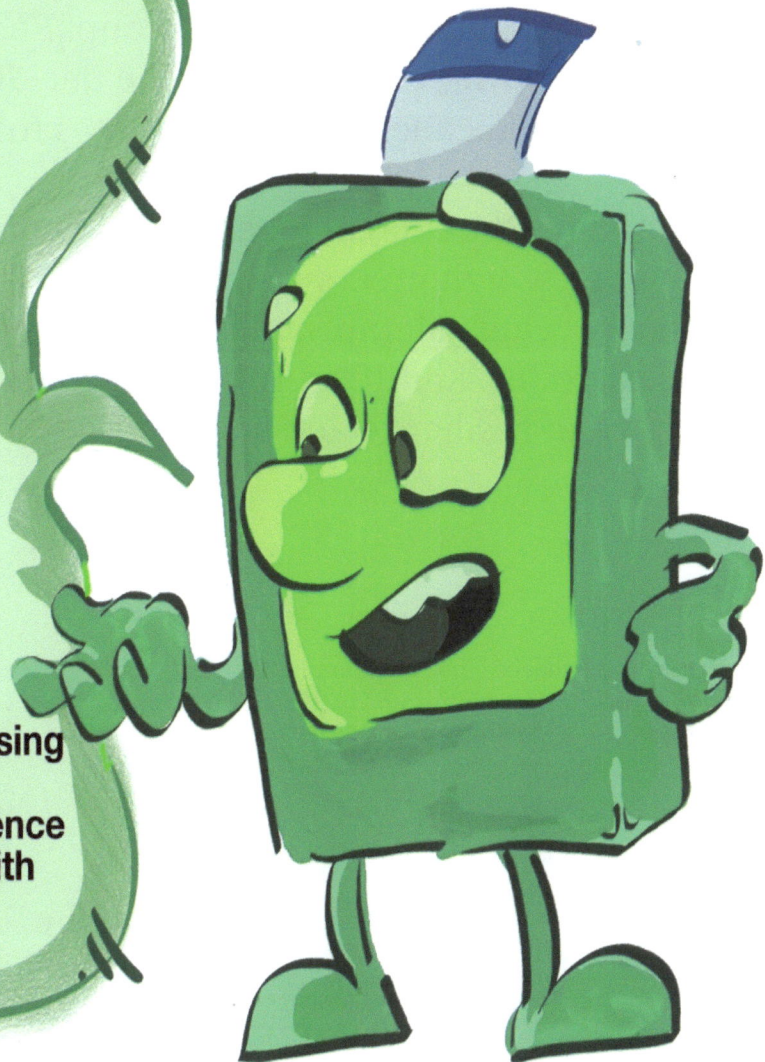

About the Author

Kaitlin Michaels is seventeen years old and a junior in high school. She was diagnosed with Type 1 diabetes at the age of nine. At the time she was diagnosed, Kaitlin could not find a book that explained all aspects of Type 1 diabetes to children in her age group. Because Kaitlin loves science, medicine, drawing, and children, she decided to write and illustrate her own book about Type 1 diabetes for school age children.

Kaitlin plays the cello and bass guitar, competes in Science Olympiad tournaments, volunteers at the Midwest regional offices of the United States Holocaust Memorial Museum, loves to read history, and draws political cartoons. Kaitlin truly believes that Type 1 diabetes has given her strength and resilience and she is indeed happily pursuing her dreams.

www.ingramcontent.com/pod-product-compliance
Lightning Source LLC
Chambersburg PA
CBHW060833270326
41933CB00002B/67